T0361570

You Gotta Eat

You Gotta Eat

Real-Life Strategies for Feeding Yourself When Cooking Feels Impossible

MARGARET EBY

Illustrated by María Toro

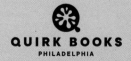

QUIRK BOOKS

PHILADELPHIA

Library of Congress Cataloging-in-Publication Data

Names: Eby, Margaret, author. | Toro, María, illustrator.

Title: You gotta eat : real-life strategies for feeding yourself when cooking feels impossible / Margaret Eby ; illustrated by María Toro.

Description: Philadelphia : Quirk Books, [2024] | Includes index. | Summary: "A guide to making easy, tasty meals when stressed, burned out, or exhausted, including meal suggestions, accessible preparation methods, and simple recipes"—Provided by publisher.

Identifiers: LCCN 2024010578 (print) | LCCN 2024010579 (ebook) | ISBN 9781683694427 (hardcover) | ISBN 9781683694434 (ebook)

Subjects: LCSH: Quick and easy cooking. | LCGFT: Cookbooks.

Classification: LCC TX833.5 .E285 2024 (print) | LCC TX833.5 (ebook) | DDC 641.5/12—dc23/eng/20240312

LC record available at https://lccn.loc.gov/2024010578

LC ebook record available at https://lccn.loc.gov/2024010579

ISBN: 978-1-68369-442-7

Printed in China

Typeset in Peanut Donuts, Kalam, and Freight

Designed by Elissa Flanigan

Cover and interior illustrations by María Toro

Quirk Books
215 Church Street
Philadelphia, PA 19106
quirkbooks.com

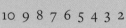

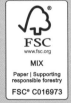

FSC
www.fsc.org
MIX
Paper | Supporting
responsible forestry
FSC® C016973

FOR KAT KINSMAN,
WHO TAUGHT ME THAT WRITING
ABOUT FOOD IS REALLY WRITING
ABOUT FEELINGS

INTRODUCTION

You Don't Have to Cook

.... 8

Open Something

.... 17

How to eat when your energy will only stretch as far as opening a can, container, or bag

Assemble Something

.... 55

How to eat when you want to get a little creative with presentation, but also use the stove as little as possible

Microwave Something

.... 87

How to eat when you're capable of cooking, but only if the cooking happens in under ten minutes and you mainly push a button

Blend Something

.... 107

How to eat when a blender or food processor is accessible but chewing sounds kinda hard

Cook Something

.... 125

How to eat when you have the wherewithal to fry, slice, chop, or mash—but not too much

CONCLUSION

Go Eat Something

.... 180

APPENDIX

Let's Talk About Groceries

.... 183

INDEX OF RECIPES.................................. 187

INDEX OF INGREDIENTS.............................. 188

ACKNOWLEDGMENTS................................... 190

Introduction

You Don't Have to Cook

Let's get this out of the way: You do not have to cook.

I like cooking, generally speaking. I am one of those kitchen nerds who have multiple kinds of salt on hand at any time. I went to culinary school, and I've worked at a fancy glossy food magazine with cover images of sumptuous dishes that take forty-eight hours to make. I have kept a sourdough starter (her name is Enya) alive for years. I've assembled a croquembouche, that most finicky of pastry creations, for fun. I have been one of those people at the other end of a cooking emergency hotline during Thanksgiving, instructing people how to best salvage their dry turkeys and underwhelming mashed potatoes.

But I'm also a human being, and like many human beings I have depression and anxiety. When I'm exhausted, depressed, burned out, or otherwise hitting a wall, there is no Martha Stewart recipe in the world that can entice me to make a finicky meal. No amount of exhorting that fresh is better matters if the idea of obtaining vegetables feels as overwhelming as biking across the Sahara without a support team. During the worst days of the COVID-19 pandemic, I was stuck inside a dinky one-bedroom apartment in Brooklyn, looking at recipes all day for my job at *Food & Wine*. I couldn't live entirely off takeout without bankrupting myself, but I simply couldn't face the idea of making myself an actual meal. I made a lot of impromptu cheese plates and peanut butter and jelly sandwiches, and I invested in a party-size bag of Bagel Bites. I was editing stories about lovingly handmade tamales that involved making your own masa—and there I was behind the screen, wrung out with anxiety, freaking out about my many family members who work at hospitals, and eating a hastily scraped-together lunch of string cheese, an apple, and a handful of stale trail mix.

It happened to me again in the winter of 2022 to 2023, this time during a depressive episode that left me struggling to extricate myself from bed, let alone figure out feeding myself. When I'm depressed, food seems so unappealing that I ignore it until I'm ravenous and angry and possibly crying. At my lowest point, sometime that January, my husband would bring me a piece of fruit and not leave the room until I put in the effort to consume it. No amount of culinary training or poring over recipes or looking at beautiful images of immaculate food was enough at that time to convince me to make anything more complicated than a grilled cheese.

Every single fancy food professional I know, from James Beard–nominated chefs to reality cooking show judges to cookbook writers to restaurant critics, has days (or months or years) like this. It's not that everyone is clinically depressed, but there are a whole host of reasons that make cooking feel like a slog: sleep deprivation, illness, busy time at work, insomnia, family emergency, having a sweet but fussy newborn, burnout, just not feeling up to it today, et cetera, et cetera. Even people who really love cooking and are really good at it have days when they eat like a cranky toddler. It's completely fine, and it's completely normal.

As a culture, though, we insist on being weird about it. Food is in a pretty unique position as human endeavors go: every person on earth has an interaction with food (or lack thereof) every single day, in all kinds of capacities. As a result, food, cooking, and feeding yourself also carry all kinds of cultural assumptions. The internet is rife with them—everyone has an opinion on the *best* way of preparing a dish (implying, if maybe never stating outright, that your way is *trash*, you *fool*). There's also no divorcing food from the diet-industrial complex and its attendant rigid ideas of acceptable body types and how to maintain or achieve them. Look at the comments of almost any popular recipe and you'll see the same battles being fought over and over about the inclusion of oil or sugar or salt, a blatant policing of everyone else's diets via little snipes about how olive oil will give you cancer (nope!) and gluten will ruin your life (only if you have a sensitivity to it!). It's enough to make you give up on the whole enterprise.

Plus, cooking isn't just about getting food into your body. It's also a domestic chore, and so it's inextricable from ideas about labor around the home and all its accompanying gender, race, and class assumptions. Who gets celebrated for cooking and who is expected to put food on the table without fanfare? I mean, you can guess. Even worse, we face a host of classist and ableist judgments about everything that makes cooking just a little easier, like minced garlic in a jar or boxed breadcrumbs or precut vegetables. (OK, it's true that jarred garlic has less flavor than fresh because it has been heated slightly, but sometimes it is simply worth losing 50 percent of garlic flavor for 100 percent less time spent mincing garlic.)

And that's not even touching on the deeper issues of our food system related to climate change, the welfare of the many laborers who pick crops and package meat, the neighborhoods in America where finding fresh food is impossible or ridiculously financially onerous, and global food insecurity. It's a lot. It's overwhelming. No wonder sometimes it's just easier to eat a spoonful of peanut butter—provided, of course, you can shut out the voices telling you that peanut butter is *bad for you* and you're buying the *wrong brand*.

For me, being gentle with myself was key for recovering some amount of joy in food, as was leaning into the times when I found myself actually enjoying something in the kitchen. When I noticed a moment when making or eating food sparked a little bit of joy or creativity, rather than resentment for the endless terrible indignity of having to feed myself, I tried to keep doing it. I microwaved shredded cheese onto tortilla chips, like I used to make for an after-school snack. I ate bowls of cereal, and sometimes I put a little cinnamon in the milk. I got really into tuna melts, a staple of my college days, and found that the small act of varying the things I put into the mashed tuna and mayo combination (Brine from a jar of pepperoncini! Hot sauce! A whole can of marinated artichokes. Beans?) activated the parts of my brain that found making food fun. Eventually, slowly, I brought myself back to cooking. But it took time, and it took being patient with my brain and my body, and it also took stocking up on meal replacement smoothies when I needed to put nutrients in my body.

When food felt like a chore, I kept reminding myself: the best food is the food that you'll eat. This is the mantra of this book. Michael Pollan famously had three rules for eating: "Eat food. Not too much. Mostly plants." That's nice for him! Here, we're gonna stop with the first one. And we're going to make it easy.

If you've ever clicked on a so-called easy recipe video and then immediately closed it when the host begins cheerfully chopping up an onion, please rest assured: I'm not talking easy for Julia Child. I mean *easy* easy. We will avoid creating more dishes to clean whenever possible. If there's a way to skip a step, we're gonna skip it. I will never assume that your pantry staples include unlimited fresh herbs, black garlic, or preserved lemon paste. I am not here to judge you, or to tell you that what you're doing is bad. I don't know your life! But if you need a hand with figuring out some strategies to make simple meals, to zhuzh up leftovers, to cook in a dorm kitchen, to find creative ways to make frozen meals taste less frozen, and just to let yourself off the hook, cooking-wise, well, that's what I'm here for. I don't believe that home cooking needs to be fussy or precise. For me, being in the kitchen can be a source of joy and experimentation and meditation. It can also be a *Groundhog Day*–level nightmare to realize *oh god, I have to make dinner again???* Both things are true—cooking is wonderful, cooking is a pain. It's a spectrum.

So depending on where you are on that spectrum and how much or how little energy you have, you can scan through this book and find a chapter that feels right. This is a tool to help you realize that you've already got the makings of a bean salad in your pantry, or show you a way to cook an egg without dirtying a(nother) pan. It's also a manifesto to remind you that food, and the effort you put into it, is value-neutral—you're not letting Ina Garten down if you have popcorn for dinner.

And once you've got those ideas in place, maybe a little bit of joy can creep back in. You are allowed to do the bare minimum to nourish yourself, but personally, I always get a tiny thrill of victory from making an easy, reasonably flavorful dish. And that moment of satisfaction is what this book is all about—making meals that are delicious and, dare I say, spiritually nourishing even when the idea of getting out a chopping board fills you with dread. It's about figuring out how to make whatever you're working with a tiny bit more exciting or palatable, while also acknowledging that at the end of the day you're just an animal who needs nutrients. The best food is the food you'll eat, but sometimes the food you're willing to eat can be made just a little more fun.

I'm writing this book because it's one that I wish I had on hand countless times. To paraphrase our national poet John Denver, some days are croquembouches, others are Triscuits dipped in cream cheese. This book is for the latter days. I hope it makes your life a little easier, or more flavorful, or simply opens your eyes to the possibility of leftover Doritos crumbs being used as a condiment. After all, you don't have to cook, but you do gotta eat.

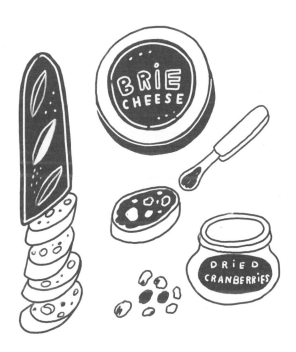

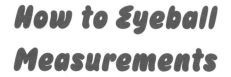

How to Eyeball Measurements

If you'd rather estimate than deal with measuring things, here are a few little tricks that can help you out.

- 1 teaspoon: roughly the size of the first joint of your thumb (from the tip of your thumb to the knuckle)
- 1 tablespoon: roughly the size of your whole thumb
- 1 cup: about the size of your fist
- ¼ teaspoon: a pinch of something grasped between your thumb and your index finger

If you don't mind dirtying dishes, but you don't own or can't bear the thought of digging out specialized measurement utensils, it's also fine to use a small spoon for a teaspoon, a big spoon for a tablespoon, and a regular coffee mug for a cup.

When you guesstimate, use nonstandard equipment, or just vibe it out, the measurements won't be as precise, but it won't matter. None of the recipes in this book—with one exception, Two-Ingredient Mug Cake (page 104)— require precision. By the same token, don't worry about having slightly more or less of what the recipe specifies. If you have a slightly smaller or larger can of chickpeas than the one I'm calling for, that's not a big deal. If a recipe calls for two tomatoes and you only have one tomato, that recipe is still going to work just fine, it'll just be a little less tomatoey. You're not going to ruin anything!

You can guesstimate when preparing recipes outside this book, too—just bear a few things in mind. One, baking does, actually and unfortunately, require precision—it's worth dirtying your tablespoons and cups, or using a kitchen scale if you have one. (Skip the scale if that feels too intimidating, but I find it easier to use and clean up than using a dozen fiddly little spoons.) Second, it's completely fine to experiment with adding or reducing amounts in a recipe, but typically I wouldn't go more than one and a half to two times the original amount. If a recipe calls for a tablespoon of lime juice and you add a cup, that is going to be extremely lime-flavored. That's not necessarily a problem if that's what you want, but it might drown out other flavors you were hoping to taste. And finally, the idea that there is no such thing as too much garlic is, sadly, a myth—ask me about the time I made a pesto that was so garlicky I could see through time.

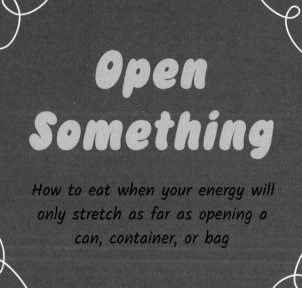

Open Something

How to eat when your energy will only stretch as far as opening a can, container, or bag

Sometimes the sum total of what I can deal with in the kitchen is popping the tabs on some cans, ripping open a box or bag, and maybe, *maybe* boiling water. If you're feeling like you just might opt to starve to death if nobody invents a way to teleport food directly into your mouth in the next forty-eight hours, this book is the place to start. We've got ways to turn canned soup into something that tastes a bit less canned, plus an easy trick to turn a jar of tomato sauce into a tomato soup. We've got ways to make your instant ramen or mac and cheese more filling and less sad, a stew you don't have to think about, the simplest of spread-it-and-forget-it sandwiches, and the ultimate open-and-dump meal: bean salad. Grab your can opener and follow me.

Bean Salad, the Musical Salad

Canned beans are beautiful. They're already cooked. They have a ton of protein and fiber. They're filling. And they're really inexpensive. You may think *salad* means "sad privation meal of lettuce," but actually salad is a loose category that roughly translates to "haphazard assembly of things tied together by dressing," and by this definition beans are the perfect vehicle. All you need to do is open them, drain them, rinse them if you have the energy but not if you don't (they might just taste slightly more metallic), dump them in a bowl, combine with dressing and perhaps other stuff, and stir. Behold: lunch.

Precut veggies (including frozen—let the salad sit for a bit after mixing to let the frozen veggies defrost) work just fine here. So do bottled dressings, though if you don't have those you can always use the time-honored classic of olive oil, vinegar, salt, and pepper (or, if you're feeling very fancy, the Nora Ephron classic of a tablespoon of dijon mustard, a tablespoon of red wine vinegar, and 3 tablespoons of olive oil, whisked together with a fork). Try one of these combinations, or get creative! The more comfortable you get in the bean salad space, the more you'll be able to branch out.

- Chickpeas + cucumbers + cherry or grape tomatoes + tzatziki = Greek-ish salad
- Black beans + thawed frozen corn + half jar of salsa + crunched-up tortilla chips = nacho salad
- Cannellini beans + pesto + parmesan = sort of Italian bean salad
- Kidney beans + celery + sweet onions + pickle relish = what if a hot dog condiment bar was a salad
- Black beans + mashed or chopped-up avocado + lime juice + hot sauce or Tajín = what if guacamole was a salad
- Chickpeas, smushed + celery + mayo + dab of dijon mustard = tuna salad without tuna
- Great northern beans + leafy greens you need to use up + balsamic vinegar + olive oil = classic house salad
- Black-eyed peas + celery + bell peppers + hot sauce + red wine vinegar + pinch of sugar/dab of honey/little bit of maple syrup = Hoppin' John–inspired salad
- Edamame + carrot + green onion + ginger dressing = teppanyaki-restaurant-inspired salad

Roll Your Own Bean Salad

If you're not sure how to start, let random chance make a salad for you. Each category has six options. Roll a die, choose an ingredient from each column, and go. (If you hate what you rolled, roll again or pick a different thing. Dice do not carry the force of law.)

BEANS

1. Edamame
2. Chickpeas
3. Pinto beans
4. Black beans
5. White beans (cannellini, great northern, etc.)
6. Black-eyed peas

VEGETABLES

1. Leafy greens
2. Corn kernels
3. Avocado
4. Cherry tomatoes
5. Chopped onion (red, white, or green)
6. Bell peppers

DRESSING

1. Olive oil and vinegar
2. Hot sauce or salsa
3. Pesto or grab-bag green sauce (page 115)
4. Green goddess dressing
5. Lime or lemon juice
6. Mayonnaise and/or mustard

EXTRAS

1. Cheese (parmesan, goat cheese, feta, etc.)
2. Crumbled tortilla chips
3. Nuts or seeds
4. Fresh herbs like parsley or cilantro
5. Cooked grains (farro, quinoa, etc.)
6. Hard-boiled egg

Anything's a Sandwich If You're Not a Coward

The first rule of sandwich club is you talk about sandwiches constantly. You never shut up about sandwiches, ideally. I could have a conversation about sandwiches and their discontents with anyone on earth, I'm pretty sure. I'm being liberal with the word *sandwich* here. A hot dog, to me, is a sandwich, and so is a taco, and so is a kathi roll, and so is that thing you made by putting leftover dumplings and lo mein into a wrap. In this house we do not gatekeep sandwiches.

The most essential part of a sandwich is its container. You do need some kind of bread or bread-like substance in order to keep the filling bounty under control. But basically, that's where it ends. If all you have is hamburger buns or English muffins or corn tortillas or those wraps that are only made of eggs somehow, that's great. Literally, if that's *all* you have, it can still be a sandwich. There's an actual thing in Great Britain called a toast sandwich, which is, yes, a slice of toast in between two slices of normal bread, with salt, pepper, and sometimes butter. That was included in an "invalid cookery" chapter in the 1861 *Book of Household Management* by Isabella Beaton. (The cooking is valid—it's *for* invalids, an out-of-date way to say "sick people.") Pros: it's cheap! Cons: it's just bread. If that appeals to you, go for it—it basically couldn't be easier, and reportedly it's weirdly good. If you want to go a step further than a bread sandwich on bread, though, read on.

Look in the fridge. What d'ya got? Obviously sliced deli meats or sliced cheese make a great sandwich. Leftover tofu, chicken, beef, salmon, or another protein? Throw it in there and add a condiment or two, plus some vegetables that are good raw if you have them. (If you have already cooked vegetables, that's amazing, go ahead and put those in there.) Lettuce and tomato are gimmes, as are arugula or spinach, but sliced radishes are also pretty nice and peppery too. But I'm guessing if you had those things on hand you would already be eating a sandwich, so let's focus on your weirder varieties, for when the pantry is bleak and leaving the house is not great.

Usually I try to have a two-ingredient contrast: something crunchy and something soft, or something sweet and something salty. That's the same principle at play in the toast sandwich, but nowadays we have the advantage of modern refrigeration technologies and produce in a can that won't give you botulism.

TOMATO AND MAYO

This is a summertime staple in Alabama, where I grew up, because it is a perfect snack and exactly the level of cooking you want to do when it's August and outside feels like a sauna. It's just sliced tomato on untoasted bread, preferably the kind of white bread that you could collapse into a giant dough ball if you squished it hard enough. Slather both slices of the bread in mayonnaise—this probably isn't the sandwich for mayo haters, because this mayo is load-bearing and nonoptional (it seals in the tomato juices, but also the fat in the mayo provides an extremely lovely counterbalance to the acid of the tomato). Then you aggressively salt and pepper the mayonnaised bread and add slices of tomato. Then you eat it. Usually over the sink, if your tomatoes are juicy enough. If you try to fancy it up—with rustic bread or torn basil or mozzarella or what have you—it makes the sandwich worse. The simplest, most dirtbag version is by far the best. It's peak eating during tomato season, but it's perfectly serviceable any time of year. But if you're deep in winter and the tomatoes are both expensive and crummy, may I suggest . . .

CANNED PINEAPPLE AND MAYO

People who follow along nodding about tomato sandwiches usually abandon ship on this one, and I get it. It's weird. It's another Southern thing, or maybe it's just a Great Depression thing. You do the same thing as with a tomato sandwich, but swap the tomato for canned pineapple (the sliced kind—chunks are OK but harder to eat and you'd probably want to cut each chunk in half for optimal thickness, which is a pain). It sounds gross! But I promise you, it's one of those three-ingredient meals that really works, thanks to the sweet acidity of the pineapple being tamed by the fat in the mayonnaise. Another classic variation of this is the banana and mayonnaise sandwich favored by racecar driver Dale Earnhardt Jr. Personally, bananas don't provide enough contrast for me, and if I have a banana around I usually integrate it into a peanut butter sandwich (see page 24) or just straight up eat a banana. But it's an option!

BUTTER AND JAM

Actual queen Elizabeth II *loved* a butter and jam sandwich with the crusts cut off. It's another three-ingredient banger, again thanks to the sweet-acid thing that the jam is laying down contrasted with the salty-fat thing that the butter is bringing to the table. (If your butter is unsalted, simply sprinkle a pinch of salt on there.) The queen's favorite jam when she didn't have homemade preserves was, allegedly, Tiptree Little Scarlet Strawberry Preserve, made from the finest and tiniest ripe strawberries. But the store-brand stuff you have hanging out works the same.

CHEESE AND JAM, CHUTNEY, OR HONEY

Boy, are you going to be sick of reading the word *acid* at the end of this, but anyway, that's the deal here too. Jam gives you some pop, cheese gives you some salt and fat and umami, and this combination works with any cheese you've got. If no jam is around (and first of all, are you *sure* no jam is around? Jams, jellies, and preserves tend to be the kinds of things that kick around a refrigerator for years, unused but basically fine), try something else that you'd find on a cheese plate—relish or chutney is great. Honey doesn't give you the same sweet-acid thing, but it's still a nice contrast to the cheese, particularly if you have a sharp, smoky, or salty cheese like cheddar or gouda.

PEANUT BUTTER AND HOT SAUCE

Ha *ha* you thought I was going to say jelly, didn't you? No. I mean yes, but you already knew about that. Peanut butter and sriracha, though—have you tried that? It works, an unholy marriage of the savory umami peanut butter and the spicy vinegary hot sauce. Try it!

PEANUT BUTTER AND APPLE (OR CELERY, OR BANANA)

I like crunchy peanut butter as much as the next person without a life-threatening allergy to it, but sometimes I want it to be even crunchier. To achieve that, I add celery or apple slices to the sandwich, which is, yes, a sandwichified version of an after-school snack. Celery seems to turn into goo within hours of getting it home from the store, so you *probably* don't have any extra lying around in a usable state, but if you've got some neglected celery that you've miraculously caught in its five good minutes, for god's sake try this before it liquifies. (Also if you have celery that has turned rubbery but not yet into goo and you want to resuscitate it, just soak it in ice water for half an hour.) I also like a banana and peanut butter sandwich, which isn't crunchy but *is* a different category of mush, and sometimes that just hits.

TOMATO PASTE AND AVOCADO

For this one I have to tip my hat to chef Kiki Aranita, who opened my eyes to the off-label use of tomato paste. She squiggles a bit of tomato paste from a tube onto her sandwiches. I tried it and I'm never going back. Tomato paste in a tube is more expensive than the canned stuff, but those teeny cans tend to get lost in my fridge and emerge weeks later infested with mold. The tube kind lets you use a little at a time, and it's often double concentrated for even more tomato flavor. Tomatoes contain natural MSG (yes! See also: mushrooms, parmesan) and so they have that great umami, why-can't-I-stop-eating-this quality. Tomato paste in the same realm as ketchup, but more intense. Spreading that onto the bread before the avocado makes the whole thing come together and feel more like a meal.

HUMMUS AND CUCUMBER OR PICKLES

Honestly, hummus alone on a sandwich is great, and something I've eaten on more than one occasion. But if you have cucumber or celery or another vegetable that's essentially crunchy water, it makes for such a lovely pairing. If you have feta around, throw it in there too. Alternatively, pickles are also crunchy water but additionally salty (no need for extra salt from feta!) and have a longer refrigerator shelf life than fresh veggies, and they work incredibly here.

CREAM CHEESE AND PICKLES OR OLIVES

I have pickles and olives on hand way, way more often than I have cucumbers because they last forever. Pickles and peanut butter is a joke about pregnancy cravings but actually it's also excellent in its own way. It's sharp and salty and smooth and creamy all at the same time. Pickles and cream cheese (or, if you want to get super fancy, cornichons dipped in crème fraîche) is a flavor sensation with everything: saltiness, creaminess, sharpness, unctuous fattiness. It's like if a cucumber and cream cheese finger sandwich was a little more rugged. It operates on the same principle as adding pickles to your cheeseburger, but without all that tedious mucking around with ground beef. It also works with basically any mild cheese: mozzarella, American, cheddar, gouda, brie, ricotta, even mascarpone if you have that instead. I haven't tried it with a ton of other cheeses but I sure would! If you don't have or like pickles, olives work too, but make sure they're pitted; otherwise, things get crunchy in a bad way.

CHIP SANDWICH

I'm sure I'm not the first person to tell you to add potato chips or corn chips to your sandwich. It's a great, easy trick—chips are salty and crunchy and delicious, and they play well inside bread. In Ireland, where my mom is from, there is a semi-famous delicacy known as a Tayto sandwich, in which you slather two slices of white bread with good butter and then crunch in a bag of Tayto cheese and onion chips. It's a desperation classic. You can do the same with any chips you have on hand, or you can add a handful of them to whatever else you're making to see how they offset the flavor. That applies to everything from a PB and J to a plain cheese sandwich to a more extravagant affair with grilled chicken or tuna salad or slivered roast beef. I personally love adding them to an otherwise extremely plain turkey and cheese. It's instant satisfaction. If you want to get fancy and thoughtful about matching up the chips to the contents of the sandwich you can, but I really have never run into a situation in which the flavors of the chip clash with the flavors of the sandwich. Just don't use a chip flavor you hate (why would you do that anyway?) and you're golden.

Most Things Can Also Be Toast

What if you don't have more than one slice of bread, or the thing you want to put into a sandwich will make it cartoonishly vertical and impossible to eat, à la Dagwood? No worries, man. Toasts are just the convertible of sandwiches.

Toasted bread is sturdier than untoasted, so it can stand up to much more. Plus, you can eat a toast with a knife and fork instead of picking it up as you would a sandwich (though you also *can* pick it up). That means you can pile on ingredients with abandon without worrying about the contents spilling out all over your clothes. And also, you can get sort of weird with it. Baked beans in a sandwich is sort of iffy. Baked beans on toast is a British bachelor classic. Leftover pasta and sauce in a sandwich is an accident waiting to happen. On toast it's a dirtbag ziti pizza, and I'm for it. In fact, if you have leftovers of basically anything that's not too liquidy, why not make Leftovers Toast? Imagine pad thai toast, or chicken tikka masala toast. It's worth a shot! Forks are for suckers.

I don't need to remind you that avocado toast is a thing, but if you're not up for babysitting an avocado, it's fully legal to use guacamole from a container. And toasts don't have to look like the architectural, Instagrammable avocado toasts on cool restaurant menus. You can just spread something on a piece of toast for a surprisingly satisfying meal. Consider: Nutella toast. Toast and butter. Toast and peanut butter (or almond butter, or sunflower seed butter, or . . .). Toast and cheese. Toast and Vegemite, if you like that kind of thing. A piece of toast plus a filling plus a slice of cheese is a melt, another great category of thing. The simplest melt is an open-faced grilled cheese, but you can also add a dab of tomato sauce or tomato paste before the cheese goes on and make pizza toast. (Even a simple grilled cheese can get complicated—people have all sorts of opinions on how to make the *best* one, and they tend to involve pans and stoves and spatulas—but you're not trying to run a diner or win a contest here, you're just trying to eat a sandwich. Just put a slice of cheese on bread and put it in the toaster oven.)

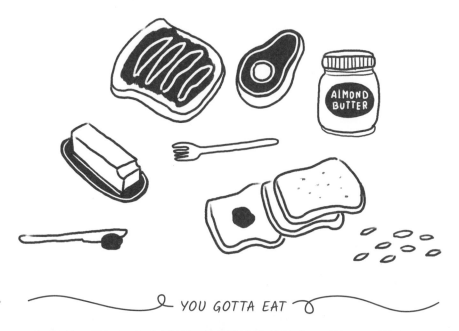

Prove It's Not Stew, I Dare You

Stew is a pretty loose concept. What is it? Basically an assemblage of random things pulled together with a broth. A salad with a liquid base, if you will. So it is a great candidate for a meal when you can't figure out quite what makes sense, and a great way to use up the weird little dribs and drabs of produce that are lingering in your fridge before they enter the dread vegetable sludge abyss. If you have a can of soup, great. That's a stew starter (especially if it already has stuff in it). All you need to do is throw in whatever you have that doesn't seem like it would be gross in a stew and voilà.

Important note: you can soup up your soup with any one of the additions below, or any two, or any five, or all of them. You are not going to make your stew worse by doing too much. And if you do too little . . . listen, it's a can of soup, the people who made it are food professionals, it will also be fine.

First, get out a pot, open a can of soup, and dump it in the pot. If it's a concentrate (check the label and instructions, they'll tell you), add water according to the instructions to avoid making an accidental hyperconcentrated salt bomb. Here's what to add to a can of soup to make it into a meal.

HERBS, DRIED OR FRESH

I told you I didn't expect you to always have fresh herbs at your disposal, and I meant it. But if you happen to have some slowly wilting in the crisper drawer, or you have an overgrown basil shrub out on the balcony or back patio, using them is a great way to brighten up canned soup. If your fresh herbs are the tender kind that can wilt easily—cilantro, basil, parsley—go nuts, add a fat handful. If they're woodier, the kind whose stem you wouldn't eat—rosemary, thyme, sage—be a little more restrained lest you end up feeling like you're eating a topiary. If you don't have fresh herbs, then dig around your spice cabinet for dried herbs like parsley, oregano, thyme, marjoram, tarragon, or sage. You *can* overdo these—counterintuitively, dried herbs are a whole lot stronger than fresh, although they might have lost some potency if they've been sitting around in your cabinet for three years, no judgment—so restrict yourself to a teaspoon or so, and you can always add more later. I've found some frozen blocks of cilantro and basil in the grocery store and those are excellent mimics for the fresh stuff. The tubes of paste work well too, and they last forever in the fridge.

MISO PASTE

Miso is incredible. It adds instant flavor depth to sauces, soups, and stews, and if you have some knocking around your fridge, you should use it (it lasts for a year in the fridge so it's likely fine!). The main thing to remember is that it's really salty, so if you're doctoring up a can of soup that's already pretty salt-heavy, be sure to go slow and taste as you go. Swirl in a teaspoon or so and see how it tastes to you—it'll work with anything you have on hand. There are several colors of miso paste with slightly different flavor profiles but any of them will be a winner.

VEGETABLES

Cans of soup often have vegetables included, but they can be pretty underwhelming. If you have leftover cooked vegetables, particularly if they're already cut into bite-size pieces, they are perfect to throw into soup. If you don't, but you have some frozen vegetables, that's great too. I like frozen peas, frozen mushrooms, or a small amount of frozen spinach here, but you can get creative. Eyeball the amount of veggies you want to add and throw them into the pot. Bring it back to a simmer and cook until the vegetables are as soft as you want them to be—just fish one out and taste it to see how it's going. How long will depend on the kind of vegetables you have and your personal kitchen conditions, but it shouldn't take more than 5 to 10 minutes, all told. This is also a good use for those greens you bought in a fit of optimism that are about to die a tragic death. If you're ready to chop a vegetable, you're probably not reading this section (there's a whole chapter later on for people with chopping energy), but I'll also add that mushrooms and asparagus can be torn or snapped by hand and cook quickly.

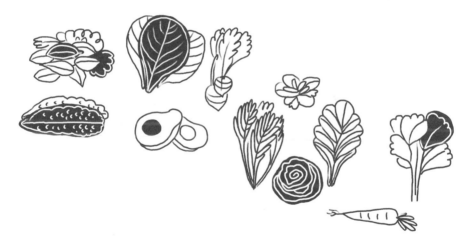

CANNED BEANS

Many soups are already bean based, for the very good reason that brothy beans are tasty and nourishing. There's something a little bit rugged and cowpoke-like about a good pot of brothy warm beans, no? Living off the *land*! And by land I mean trusty corner bodega. Adding beans to a can of soup ups the protein content and brings a little more fiber to the whole affair, meaning it'll keep you full for longer. If you want a stew to be thicker, mash the beans right in the can with a fork before you add them to the pot.

LENTILS

Lentils are the adorable, inexpensive, quick-cooking cousins of Big Bean, and they're just great in stews. They come dried in bags, not cooked in a can like beans, so you'll need to cook them into the soup for a little longer, but just 20 to 30 minutes. The good news is that the process is extremely hands-off. Literally grab a fistful of lentils (or pour them into the cup of your hand) and throw them in.

Brown and green lentils tend to collapse into the surrounding broth and give the whole bowl a subtle earthiness. Yellow and red lentils, my favorite, break down into absolute mush—they're often used in dal. If you add them to a premade can of soup, follow the directions on the bag and add some more water so they can cook down into it (fill your empty soup can with water and dump that in). Don't worry about the stew being too diluted—as the lentils cook, they'll absorb the water and release starch, which will make the whole thing come together.

One of my favorite go-to winter depression meals, one that evolved from a recipe by Chef Yotam Ottolenghi, is a can of crushed tomatoes, a tablespoon of curry powder, ½ cup of red lentils, 2 cups of water, and a can of coconut milk, all cooked together until it turns into beautiful stew mush, roughly half an hour. It's incredible with Tostitos Hint of Lime chips (or any similarly flavored tortilla chips) or a dollop of sour cream or yogurt on top, and absolutely everything in it is shelf-stable enough to survive an apocalypse.

SPLASH OF VINEGAR OR LEMON JUICE

Look, this is not the last time I'm going to tell you how magical acid is. Particularly if the soup you have is dairy based—chowder, cream of mushroom, cheese and broccoli, bisque, et cetera—the zip that comes from a splash of vinegar or squeeze of lemon is really going to liven that sucker up. But any soup benefits from a splash of acid. Chicken noodle soup with a little bit of lemon juice, or even pickle brine? Heaven.

LEFTOVER PROTEIN

Do you have meat that's already cooked in the fridge? Like, what's that over there—a rotisserie chicken hanging out? Shred some meat and plop it in. Leftover ham? Cut it into li'l ham cubes and add. Ground turkey? Sure, yes. Leftover sausage is honestly ideal. A sprinkling of cooked crispy bacon on top is an instant enhancement. That'll bulk that soup right up.

LITTLE PASTA

Another great way to bulk up canned soup, particularly if the soup isn't already noodle based, is to add some teeny pastas. The best ones for this purpose are guys that are bite-size and cook quickly, like orzo, ditalini, pastina, or fideo. (Fideo is just broken-up spaghetti, so if you have spaghetti, you've got fideo.) Cook the pasta directly in the soup, and it should release its precious, delicious starch and slightly thicken the liquid. Small amounts of uncooked pasta become *large* amounts of cooked pasta, so start with an amount that fills the cup of your hand. If you use too much you may wind up with more of a saucy pasta dish than a stew, but is that so bad? (If you've overdone it and you want it to be soup again, just add some more water or broth, or you could even toss some wine in there.)

CRUNCHY THINGS ON TOP

Adding some textural contrast to a soup or stew is a great way to make it feel a little more complete. All the traditional soup toppings are fair game here—oyster crackers, croutons, mini butter crackers—but don't discount other crunchies that might be knocking around, like crumbled-up chips, the fried noodles from Chinese takeout, wasabi peas, Cheetos, crispy chickpeas, and coconut chips. Don't worry too much about flavors that "match" or "go together"—if it tastes good to you outside of soup, it will probably taste good on top of soup. (Caveat: when the purpose is crunch, steer away from things that famously get soggy quickly. I once put Cheerios on top of a stew and I can't really recommend it, despite the prevailing theory that cereal is a kind of breakfast soup.)

Do Exactly This: Tomato Sauce Soup

So you want soup but what you have is a jar of tomato sauce, like the kind you use on spaghetti. But what if I told you that tomato soup . . . is just thinned-out tomato sauce?

It's true. It's real! Your sauce can convert into a soup. A standard size jar of tomato sauce makes roughly four bowls.

Ingredients
- Olive oil (one or two glugs)
- 1 jar tomato sauce

- The same amount of **stock** or **broth** or **water**
- Salt and pepper

Optional
- Red pepper flakes
- Dried oregano or an Italian-type spice blend
- Worcestershire sauce or red wine vinegar
- ½ to 1 cup cream
  - If you don't have cream, **half-and-half** or whole milk
  - If you don't have or want half-and-half or whole milk, a **milk alternative** like oat milk, almond milk, soy milk, or coconut milk
- ½ cup grated **hard cheese**, like parmesan or pecorino

1. Splash some olive oil in stock pot (or any big pot you'd use for soup), enough that it makes a thin layer that coats the bottom. Heat it on medium until the oil starts shimmering, or just until you sense that, yeah, that pot is getting hot.
2. Dump in your jar of tomato sauce. Fill that same jar with stock, broth, or water. Then add that. Stir it in, and then taste the mixture. If it still veers more toward sauce, add more liquid (just use water if you used all your stock or broth. Let the mixture come to a simmer.
3. Once it seems like the right consistency and is simmering merrily, then you can season it if you want! Add a few shakes or grinds of black pepper or red pepper flakes or some of that oregano or Italian seasoning. A teaspoon or so of

Worcestershire sauce is nice, or a teaspoon or two of red wine vinegar. (You can use the spoon you're going to eat with to measure this, it's not that finicky.) Every time you add something, stir it in and then taste the soup—that way, you can adjust the ingredients accordingly.

4. If you don't have any dairy then you can stop here. If you do, it's nice to add some to the soup to give it a velvety texture. Add about ½ cup cream, half-and-half, whole milk, or plant milk, and stir it in. Does the mixture taste too sharp? Add more dairy. Does it taste sort of flat? Add more salt. If it's too sweet, add more vinegar. If you have grated parmesan or pecorino, sprinkle it in a little at a time, stirring all the while to integrate the cheese into the soup. Start with a little bit, taste, and add until you like how it's going.

5. When the mixture tastes like tomato soup to you, it's done! Top it with something crunchy if you want, or put more cheese or a dollop of sour cream on top if you've got some. You did it. It's soup.

A Spice Manifesto

Spices are useful and powerful ingredients, but they can be intimidating to use. I get it. You don't want to add way too much of something and ruin a dish, or make something so overwhelmingly spicy that the only option is to throw it out and defrost some chicken nuggets. But I am here to say that you should use the contents of your spice cabinet both liberally and weirdly. If you have an idea for a spice that might go well in something, then go for it. If you have no idea, but you have all these spices around so you might as well use them, also go for it.

The trick is to start slow. Stir or sprinkle a pinch—like a literal pinch, just pick it up with your (clean) fingers—into whatever you're making and try it. If you like the flavor, add more. As long as you add them incrementally, even strong spices shouldn't get too overwhelming. But if you do go too far, don't worry! You can rescue an overspiced dish by adding dairy or some acid, like a splash of vinegar or a squeeze of lemon juice, to round out the flavors a little bit.

Chili, a Stew with Dreams

Chili is a subset of soups and stews, but it's really its own thing, much as Texas is technically part of the United States but also functionally its own distinct nation. The mention of Texas here is not casual—chili is one of those dishes that make people get incredibly heated about what does and doesn't belong in it, and Texans tend to feel especially strongly. In fact, if you're from Texas you may want to skip this section. You don't want to half-ass chili. Back up and make a stew.

There are those who believe—again, Texans primarily—that a good bowl of chili has no beans in it. There are whole competitive cookoffs devoted to fighting over the essential nature of chili, and lord knows I am not the arbiter of what counts. I am the arbiter of what you can shove in your face with no effort when you need to eat something, and chili—not cookoff-winning chili, maybe not Texan-approved chili, but chili nonetheless—is one of the greats.

There are many, many articles on the easiest way to make chili, whether that's in an electric pressure cooker or a slow cooker or in a stockpot. But they're all incorrect: the easiest way to make chili is just to buy it in a can, dump the can into a pot, and heat it up. Chili in a can has many virtues, namely, that it's already made for you and can live in your pantry for years, just waiting for the day when you pop it open. But usually it could use a little bit of help in the flavor and texture departments. Luckily, it is wildly easy to give canned chili a bit of extra oomph without much effort.

ADD BEER (OR WINE)

You know how I'm always talking about acid? Beer and wine are acidic—wine more so than beer—which means that they can add contrast and a little pop of brightness to your chili without a lot of effort.

Beer is a classic addition to chili because of the malty notes and bitterness, both things that can add a bit more flavor complexity to the mix. If you don't have beer but you do have wine, a cup of it will also bring out more flavor. Red wine is particularly great for this, but you can use whatever you have. I'd avoid super-sweet wines, such as moscatos, because I don't love very sweet chili, but you do you. When you dump your can of chili into a pot, add a can of beer or a glass of wine. Bring the whole thing to a simmer, which will cook off the alcohol but leave the flavor, which means you can drink another beer with your chili if you want to.

STIR IN COCOA POWDER

Chocolate and beef or beans seems like a weird mixture, but cocoa powder is a secret ingredient in so many family chili recipes for a reason. Think about how it works in a great mole sauce to kind of anchor the other spices and give them a great underlying bitterness. Find some unsweetened cocoa powder, like the kind you'd use for making brownies, and stir a teaspoon (or just a dash if you're trepidatious) into the chili. It'll make things pop.

THROW IN SPICES

Chili in a can is usually pretty mild in the spice department. It's easy to fix that by stirring in some of what you have knocking around your pantry. There's honestly not many spices that chili cannot accommodate, even if they aren't traditionally used. That's the beauty of chili! Just add a little, stir it, taste it, and see how it is. A teaspoon of cumin or smoked paprika will make things earthier, and a little cinnamon is a nice little booster (just don't add a huge amount or it'll make your chili taste like Christmas). It's not going to surprise you that chili powder is a good addition to chili, but I had to say it anyway. If you have something spicy, like red pepper flakes, dried peppers, or harissa, adding a bit to the canned chili can coax out the other flavors too. Hot sauce is great because it adds heat as well as acid to the mix. A sprinkle of onion powder or garlic powder also doctors up the flavors in chili nicely.

ADD SALSA

If you ask a chef how to make a can of chili good, they're going to tell you to add fresh vegetables. While that is a valid and reasonable response, I didn't get into the canned chili game because I want to chop things. If you do, then go for it—cilantro or chopped raw onions, celery, or carrots would all be great. But if you're like, *man, I would love to have a little bit more vegetable content in here but I am absolutely not up for finding a cutting board and a knife*, may I reintroduce you to a jar of salsa? Salsas usually have the things that taste good in a chili, like raw tomato and onion, and you don't have to do any work. To your pot of chili, add a couple tablespoons of store-bought salsa and stir it in. If you want more, you can add up to the whole jar.

GRAB SOME PICKLED JALAPEÑOS

Like salsa, pickled jalapeños are the answer to the question: how do you get the brightness and crunch of fresh vegetables without having to cut up fresh vegetables? Easy. In addition to adding a bit of spice, pickled jalapeños add some needed crunch and brightness to canned chili. You can use them as a topping, or tip in some of the pickled peppers with their liquid to the pot with the chili and stir it around.

USE THE VINEGAR AND BROWN SUGAR TRICK

When I'm making a big pot of dried beans from scratch, I usually cook the beans without much seasoning and then, at the end, add whatever I want to spice them with. That almost always includes two easy ingredients—a small amount (around ½ tablespoon) of brown sugar and a splash of apple cider vinegar. The combination of the lift from the vinegar and a little sweetness from the brown sugar really does something magical to beans. And since beans are a major component of many canned chilis, it follows that this combo would work just as well there. If your brown sugar is caked together, as most people's brown sugar is, just chip off a small chunk (it'll dissolve in the hot chili eventually) or heat it in the microwave under a damp paper towel for about 20 seconds before adding it to the pot.

ADD SOME BACON, WHY NOT?

Obviously if you don't eat bacon, skip this step. But if you do, and you happen to have some kicking around your fridge, you can cook a few strips (do NOT get out a pan! Do it in the microwave! Go to page 102 for more complete instructions) and crumble them over your chili. The bacon's fat and salt give the canned chili more lusciousness, and you get a bit more protein and heft too.

CHIP CRUMBS FOREVER

If you've never had the pleasure of having a Frito pie, let me clue you in. It's a casserole that's basically chili in a dish covered in Fritos. It can also be a great bar snack, in which a dollop of chili gets thrown into a bag of Fritos and then you use the chips to scoop up the chili and eat it. Chips are just made for chili, so if you have some around—

particularly the crumbs from the bottom of a bag of tortilla chips or corn chips—sprinkle them on top of your canned chili. Or put your canned chili on top of them like a beautiful piece of salmon on a bed of greens. Or mix them into your chili.

Do Exactly This: Throw-Everything-in-a-Pot Chili

If you want to feel that you've put in a *little* more effort than just "chili from a can" without actually putting in much more effort than chili from a can, have you considered: chili from *several* cans? All you really need to do is open up various chili-related cans and jars and throw the contents into a pot to simmer. This is what Pinterest calls a *dump meal* because, you know, you just get a bunch of stuff and dump it in. Because of scatological connotations of *dump meal,* I prefer the term *throw everything in a pot meal,* which I understand is not as catchy.

When I'm in the mood for Throw-Everything-in-a-Pot Chili, I make it vegetarian, because ground beef is not something I want to deal with. You can easily make this a not-vegetarian chili by opening another can of no-beans chili (the Texans made this). This is absolutely the kind of meal you can start in a slow cooker in the morning rather than making it in a pot at night, but I am not a morning person and never will be, so any attempt at meal prep I do before work is pretty lackluster. You could also make this in an electric pressure cooker—just throw everything in and set it to pressure-cook on high for 10 minutes. You can sub in whatever beans you have and skip the green chilis if you don't like them or prefer a milder chili. If you have a wild notion to throw something into the pot, I say go cowboy on it.

Ingredients

- 1 can **black beans**, drained
- 1 can **pinto beans**, drained (if you have a colander or strainer, you can drain both cans of beans into it together; otherwise, just try to pour off the liquid from the cans)
- 1 14.5-ounce can **diced tomato** (fire-roasted if you can get it, but plain is fine)
- 1 4-ounce can **diced green chilis**
- 1 16-ounce jar **salsa** (whatever spice level you prefer)
- 1 cup **frozen corn** (or 1 can corn, drained and rinsed)
- 2 cups vegetable, chicken, or beef **broth** (bouillon is fine)
  - If you don't have broth, 1 cup **water** and 1 cup **beer** or **wine**
  - If you don't have beer or wine, 2 cups **water**
- As many of these as you've got:
  - 1 tablespoon **chili powder**
  - 1 teaspoon **cumin**
  - 1 teaspoon **garlic powder**
  - 1 teaspoon **cocoa powder**
  - 1 tablespoon **apple cider vinegar**
  - **Salt and pepper**

Optional

- Hot sauce
- Crumbled corn chips

1. Get out a large stockpot, one big enough to boil spaghetti. Dump in all the ingredients except the vinegar and hot sauce (if you're using them) with 2 big pinches of salt and a good amount of pepper—say 10 cranks or so of the mill if you have one of those pepper mills, or 20 shakes.

2. Heat over high until the mixture begins to boil, and then lower the heat until it's just simmering—there should be a steady stream of smallish bubbles in the pot. Let it simmer for 20 minutes so the flavors have a chance to meld.

3. Add the apple cider vinegar and a dash or two of hot sauce, if you're using that. Taste it. Add salt and pepper as needed, and taste again. Add more hot sauce, vinegar, or chili powder, if you want.

4. When the chili is seasoned to your liking, scoop it into bowls and, if desired, top with crumbled chips.

Cup o' the Ramen to Ya

Instant ramen is basically a two-word synonym for "meal that's inexpensive and easy." It's the savior of college students, hungover people, and broke office workers everywhere, and a great thing to have on hand for when you need to eat *something* but the idea of doing anything harder than boiling water is too much. Like boxed mac and cheese, it's a whole separate category from the lovingly made bowls of ramen you can get at restaurants. And like boxed mac, it's a thing that's wonderful as is—but also extremely easy to spruce up, if you want something that's as simple as the instant version but with all the fun of the well-crafted restaurant meals.

It's so easy, in fact, that there's an entire category of TikTok videos devoted to instant ramen hacks, various instructions for noodle transformation that range from "not that complicated" to "chef school shit." I'm going to assume that you don't want to turn your ramen noodles, that simplest of foods, into something requiring a multistep cooking process. But I don't know your life, so if I'm wrong, there're a ton of ideas on the internet for how to use instant ramen as an ingredient in a more involved recipe. Go find them! If I'm right, though, stay here—you can easily add a few things to your instant ramen to bring in some extra flavor without extra effort.

Add spices or some easy extra protein, or try some crunchies on top (crumble up some uncooked ramen noodles on top of your cooked ramen noodles and thank me later). You can also add one of the three-ingredient sauces on page 122 rather than the flavor packet if you'd like. Buffalo ramen is very good and very easy, and you can even crumble blue cheese on top if you have some. Green goddess or ranch ramen noodles? I haven't had either, but I'd be very willing to try. Following are some ramen-specific ways to, in the words of Emeril Lagasse, kick things up a notch. This is far from a comprehensive list, but it will give you someplace to start.

PUT A SLICE OF AMERICAN CHEESE ON TOP

Yes, of course, you could make a cheese sauce with a roux and milk—or, well, *one* could—but I'm a trained chef and I still don't always have the wherewithal or the willpower to do that, nor do I always have unspoiled milk. But you know what kind of cheese basically turns into a sauce all by itself, without extra intervention from you? Good old individually wrapped slices of American cheese, which contain an ingredient called sodium citrate that helps the cheese melt evenly. You can buy a bag of sodium citrate from Amazon, so if you want to feel like a mad scientist in the kitchen, you can bring this melting magic to other kinds of cheese—add a little sodium citrate to boiling water and then throw in handfuls of fancier grated cheese for a ridiculously good queso, for instance. Experimental cheese sauces were a major staple of my meals during COVID-era quarantine. But I can't stress enough that you do not need to do this. All you need to do is pick up some sliced American cheese and heat it up—say, by sticking a slice on top of your bowl of hot, cooked instant ramen. It'll melt into a satisfying sauce and you won't even have to learn how to pronounce *roux*. This is particularly good with spicy ramen.

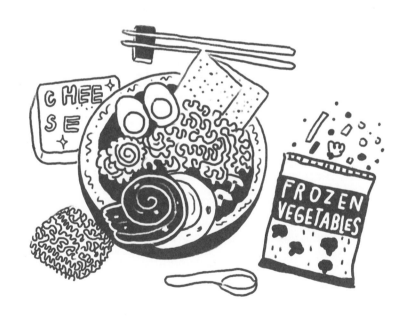

ADD AN EGG TO THE WATER

If you already have boiling hot water, then, brother, there's no reason you can't cook other things in it. Crack an egg into the hot water and noodles. Cook it for 6 to 8 minutes, 6 if you like it runnier and 8 if you like it more hard-boiled. It'll be like a poached egg in there if you just let it hang out and simmer. If you scramble it into the noodles and water, it'll cook much faster, and it'll give the whole thing a kind of egg drop soup vibe. Either way it's a little bit of extra protein and deliciousness.

ADD PEANUT BUTTER AND HOT SAUCE

If you haven't encountered this combo before, you are probably giving me a *look* right now—peanut butter on ramen noodles? But would you be giving me that look if instead of being your humble guide to the world of low-energy cooking, I were a restaurant chef? Chances are you know (and love) sesame noodles and the peanut sauces common in American Thai food—think of this as an homage to those dishes. Add 1 or 2 tablespoons of peanut butter to just-cooked ramen noodles and then add a little bit of hot sauce or chili crisp to make a savory-spicy sauce. If you don't want it to be spicy, add a splash of lime juice or vinegar instead. The heat from the noodles or broth (you can drain the noodles or not, according to your whims) will sauce-ify the peanut butter, so all you have to do is stir. This is particularly good with green onions on top, if you have any of those knocking around your fridge (just chop them into the bowl with scissors), but you don't need them.

ADD FROZEN VEGETABLES

This is the same principle as adding an egg—if you already have boiling water for the noodles, you can cook other things in there. Add a handful of frozen vegetables to the pot before you add the noodles, then bring the water back up to a boil and add the noodles. By the time the noodles are done cooking, the vegetables should be warmed through, too. This works particularly well with small vegetables like peas, edamame, and corn, though I like it with spinach, too.

CARBONARA IT

Ramen makes a great template for an easy riff on carbonara, a.k.a. bacon and eggs in noodle form. Just add an egg to the noodles, either fried (or microwaved, see page 99) or dropped right into the hot ramen broth. Then sprinkle some cooked bacon, fried Spam, or cubes of ham on top. (You can also microwave the bacon—see page 102—but we're busy people and this is best done when you have leftover cooked meat.) Add a good sprinkling of parmesan and black pepper in there, and stir it all up.

ADD MISO PASTE AND BUTTER

I will not disparage the good name of flavor packets in ramen, but there are times when you want something different. Rather than add the seasoning included with the noodles, stir a spoonful of miso paste and a tablespoon or so of butter into the boiling water when the noodles are just about cooked (in other words, when you would normally add the flavor dust). The miso adds the same salty umami notes that the flavor packet does, and the butter smooths it all out.

MAKE IT INTO RAMEN LASAGNA

Yes, I saw this on TikTok, boon to depressed chefs everywhere, and yes, I tried it and it works. It's less a lasagna in a traditional sense and more a pile of noodles baked together, but honestly, who doesn't like a pile of noodles? Take two bricks of dried ramen, a jar of pasta sauce, and some kind of cheese—ricotta or mozzarella are ideal, but I made this with a Mexican cheese blend and it was extremely delicious. All you do is take a bowl or little casserole dish and put a puddle of pasta sauce in the bottom. Then put in your brick of ramen, cover with more pasta sauce, and add a generous layer of cheese. Put another ramen brick on it, cover with more sauce, and then sprinkle on more cheese. Bake at 350°F—I used my toaster oven—for 30 to 35 minutes. Easy faux lasagna for all your Garfield cosplay needs.

Mac and Cheese and More

Every time the subject of boxed macaroni and cheese comes up, some wiseacre who has watched a lot of *Top Chef* has to pipe up to say that making macaroni and cheese without a box isn't that hard. But I have too much respect for you to parrot back that line. Could you make mac and cheese from scratch without too much trouble? Yeah, sure, you could. But boxed mac and cheese is its own thing, spiritually similar but not the same as other macaroni and cheese, like how a Taco Bell craving can't be satisfied by the lovely hole-in-the-wall taquería down the street. It's a whole separate category. In this house, we respect boxed mac and cheese.

That doesn't mean that you always have to follow the instructions on the back of the box to the letter, though. Far from it. A box of macaroni and cheese is excellent by itself, but it can also be a jumping-off point for a totally satisfying low-effort meal. Adding a can of tuna to the mix, for example, is a classic desperation American dish that would horrify most Italians. Every year, my husband's family makes a Christmas Eve dish involving several boxes of macaroni, and rather than adding water or milk to the cheese sauce, they mix in a container of sour cream, a container of tomato soup concentrate, and many handfuls of grated cheese. It might sound like one of those gross retro recipes that periodically go viral, but it's good—an ersatz tomato cream sauce with a satisfying tang from the sour cream.

If you are in a place where boxed macaroni and cheese is in your future but you want it to be a little different than the usual, here are a few ways to mix it up.

Dump it in a casserole dish: Cook the macaroni for about 2 minutes shy of what the instructions recommend, make the cheese sauce as usual, and then dump the mixture into a casserole dish. If you feel ambitious, mix in more cheese. Top it with breadcrumbs, and put it in a 450°F oven for 5 to 10 minutes until it looks crispy and good.

Throw in some spices: You know what's amazing in mac and cheese? Old Bay seasoning. You could also use taco seasoning or cajun seasoning or chili powder. A packet of ranch seasoning sort of hits—it sounds weird, but try it. It gives the same vibe as mixing together Cool Ranch and Nacho Doritos. Red pepper flakes are excellent. Adding a whole bunch of black pepper gives the dish a kind of cacio e pepe vibe. I'd steer away from stuff you might put in a dessert (although a little cinnamon might not go amiss?), but otherwise any flavor you like will probably work pretty well.

Add more dairy: We're talking about butter. We're talking about a couple solid dollops of cream cheese or sour cream. Obviously ricotta or mascarpone, for sure, yes. Cottage cheese, oh, yes. Even Greek yogurt works just fine. Whipping cream, yes, please. Swirl a couple spoonfuls into the sauce for more richness. You can also crumble in more cheese, if you like. American cheese is the superior cheese for this purpose because of how easily it turns from a solid to a sauce, so chunks of Velveeta or some crumbled American cheese works great. But if you turn your nose up at American cheese (reconsider) or simply don't have any on hand (reasonable), stir in shredded cheese like cheddar, monterey jack, pepper jack, mozzarella, or whatever blend you have. The trick is to do it a little bit at a time so it has a chance to melt, or you may end up with a brick of grated cheese on top of your macaroni. Not the worst outcome! But not what we're looking for, either.

Add condiments: Some people swear by adding ketchup to mac and cheese, and that is their journey, and I support and affirm them. I don't love ketchup on my mac—too sweet—but I will add a dollop of tomato paste sometimes. Other great things to throw in? A spoonful of spicy mustard or a smattering of chili crisp. Hot sauce is a beautiful addition. Kimchi with macaroni and cheese is incredible. Experiment and you might be surprised.

Frozen peas: That's it, that's the advice. Add frozen peas. They cook in basically the time it takes you to stir them into the pasta. They add those nice little pops of sweetness, and you also have some vegetables in there.

Easy meats: Cubed, fried Spam is an extremely good way to bulk up boxed mac and cheese and add a little textural contrast while you're at it. If you happen to have some bacon on hand, crumbling it into the mac is also incredible. Ditto rotisserie chicken or, yes, a can of tuna. Don't use the fancy kind—we're talking chunk light in water, drained and plopped right in there.

Crunchies on top: Even if you don't want to dirty a casserole dish, browning a handful of breadcrumbs in a skillet with olive oil and then dumping them on top of the mac is a delicious way to upgrade the meal. I also love sprinkling crispy fried onions from a jar, the kind that usually top green bean casseroles during Thanksgiving, on top of mac and cheese. If I've been to H Mart lately, I've probably also acquired a giant vat of fried shallots, which I'll put on everything, including noodles. Crumbled-up chips also work well here and add some extra flavor.

MACARONI OUTSIDE THE BOX

If you find yourself needing the experience of boxed macaroni and cheese but your cupboard has only noodles and no handy and delicious packets of instant cheese sauce, don't worry. (And in case this is a recurrent problem, know that you can buy a canister of the cheese sauce powder online for emergencies.) There are a couple of quick and easy ways to make cheese sauce. Could you just throw a handful of shredded cheese on the warm noodles and work with it that way? Sure you could. But if you want something that mimics the texture of boxed mac and cheese, try one of these easy techniques.

Grated cheese + pasta water: If you make a lot of pasta, you've probably heard of the idea of hanging on to some of the pasta water to make a sauce with. If you haven't, the basic concept is that the water picks up the starch from the pasta as it boils and therefore is a great way to emulsify things into a sauce. All you need to do is scoop 1 cup of pasta water from the pot before you drain your macaroni (or pasta shape of your choice). Then get a pile of grated cheese—finely grated cheese like parmesan or pecorino is ideal, but you can use whatever you have. Drain your macaroni and add it back to the pot over low heat, and have your pasta water and cheese handy. Add about ¼ cup of the pasta water to the macaroni and a handful of cheese, and stir furiously. Like, really do not relent until the cheese and water come together. Then repeat until you have sauciness to your liking.

American cheese + milk: If you have some American cheese, well, you're in luck. That stuff loves to melt. Cut or tear it into small pieces. Add a splash of milk or heavy cream—roughly ¼ cup—to the pot of cooked and drained noodles, keeping the pot over low heat. Then add your cheese pieces and stir, stir, stir. The American cheese should melt into the milk and turn into a sauce. If it's too thick, add a little bit more milk. If it's not cheesy enough, well, add more cheese. That's it.

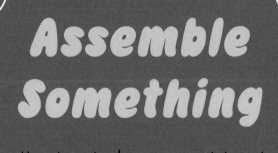

Assemble Something

How to eat when you want to get a little creative with presentation, but also use the stove as little as possible

*T*he difference between a meal and a bunch of random stuff you find in your fridge can be as simple as presentation. Loose bread and a jar of peanut butter doesn't look like a meal—but slap them together and that's a sandwich. A pile of cheese cubes and ham when spread out nicely on a plate turns into a cheese and charcuterie board. This is the chapter for you if you have a lot of things that *could* be a meal floating around, but the gentle domestic alchemy that turns ingredients to coherent dinner eludes you. We have sandwiches, of course, and also the close cousins of sandwiches: quesadillas, toasts, and snacking boards. We have dips, we have canapés, and we have nachos, the ultimate answer for when you don't know what to make but you have a bunch of chips around. Just don't forget to hang on to those leftover chip crumbs—we'll be using those later.

Mood (Cheese) Board

A cheese board contains multitudes. It can be an artful plank draped with fine charcuterie and expensive cheeses, filled in with pockets of dried fruit, nuts, olives, and jams. It can look like an Instagram dream, spread across a marble counter or a pool deck. It can also be a conference-level arrangement of cubed cheese and baby carrots with ranch and perhaps some saltines and salami somewhere in there. You can curate the cheeses by milk type, or texture, or regional affiliation, if you want to get nerdy with it. Fancy little cheese knives and marble boards and little pinch pots of jam and salt are all welcome. Esoteric crackers, Marcona almonds, and plump little dried apricots are wonderful. But those things aren't at all necessary, and if they intimidate you or make compiling a board dinner seem hard, skip them. You don't need to notify Instagram about any potential cheese board violations.

If you're just looking to make a meal pretty quickly, a cheese board can also be, as the internet would say, an adult Lunchable. Rather than assembling a sandwich or some finger bites, you just kind of let it all out there on a plate or cutting board. A cheese board for one is a great dinner. A cheese board for a group is a nice graze-y kind of meal, one that allows everyone to choose their own combinations of elements. It really can be as simple as putting some hunks of cheese onto a plate with a knife and some crackers, but it can also be scaled up or down depending on what things you have knocking around your house.

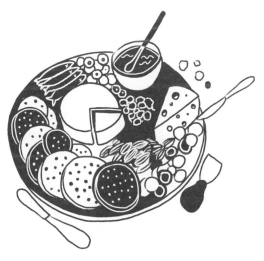

CHEESE BOARD, HOLD THE CHEESE (AND THE BOARD)

Cheese isn't even an essential ingredient—boards have no gods and no masters. Variety is encouraged, as is novelty, and all that really matters is the spirit of joyful chaos: we're not cooking, we're just compiling. As the good people of TikTok have proved on multiple occasions, you can arrange almost anything you want on a board and call it a day. A tinned fish board is great, set out with crackers and maybe some hot sauce, olives, and nuts. A charcuterie board is swell, too, and can include cheese as a minor player. You can lay out a heaping pile of lox and have some capers, cream cheese, and crackers at the ready. A board with an arrangement of cut-up fruit and vegetables, perhaps with a dip or two, is equally as dreamy. Tater tots or french fries with many dips all laid out counts as a board. Don't feel hindered if you don't have an element that's on a typical board, just root around in your pantry and fridge for what you have.

In fact, sorry to blow your mind, but you definitely don't even need a board. I like to arrange things on a cutting board, but you can make a cheese (or whatever) board on a plate, or a baking sheet, or a mirror, or directly on your counter if you really feel like cleaning very thoroughly before and after.

CHEESE BOARD ESSENTIALS

If that's not enough direction for you, I understand. The problem with an "anything goes" approach is that sometimes we get choice paralysis. If you're overwhelmed, there are some gentle principles you can follow for constructing a satisfying cheese or charcuterie board, which should also help you organize what you're pulling out of the kitchen for assembly. Here are some elements of a great board meal.

Something salty

This can include a nice hunk of a hard cheese, or it can be a purely non-cheese accompaniment. But on the whole something savory and salty—not a huge salt bomb, but something that scratches that salt-tooth itch—is a needed element on the board. Some suggestions:

- Aged cheddar
- Parmesan
- Pecorino
- Grana Padano
- Pickles or cornichons
- Olives
- Capers
- Anchovies
- Sardines
- Pistachios
- Almonds
- Blue cheese
- Salami
- Soppressata
- Prosciutto
- Mortadella
- Cashews

Something to scoop with

It is legal to just eat cheese with your hands, but it's best cheese board practice to have a foundation for building your little bites. Traditionally this is some kind of cracker, bread, or chip—but it doesn't have to be! If you're gluten-free or just don't like bready things, try rice cakes (the thin dry kind), or even thin slices of raw cucumber or carrot.

- Whole grain crackers
- Triscuits or other shredded wheat crackers
- Club crackers
- Water crackers
- Breadsticks
- Rye bread slices
- Pita chips
- Baguette slices
- Potato chips
- Rice crackers
- Corn chips

Something to spread or dip

Not only is this category a good supplement to the cheese board in general, it also provides ways to stick things to your cracker, bread, or scooping material of choice. Try:

- Cream cheese
- Butter
- Easy yogurt dip (see page 71)
- Soft cheese (like brie or goat cheese)
- Any nut butter
- Crème fraîche or sour cream
- Hummus
- Labneh
- Tuna salad or egg salad

Something sweet

Although optional, these are nice contrasts to the salty and creamy elements of the board. Consider:

- Chutney
- Jam
- Honey
- Grapes
- Dried apricots
- Dates
- Prunes
- Raisins
- Figs, dried or fresh
- Yogurt-covered pretzels

Sandwiches 2: Sandwich Harder

Yes, we already had a whole section about sandwiches. But those were sandwiches that only required you to open a jar and spread something on bread. Here, we have slightly more advanced preparation techniques. But we're still in the realm of very easy sandwiches, I promise. I am not going to suddenly ask you to sous vide something, or make your own bread, or follow any of the other time-consuming, finicky recipe directions that sometimes accompany a very good sandwich. For this, you merely need to be willing to locate a cutting board and a sharp knife, and maybe operate a toaster oven, skillet, or oven. If that's too much for where you're at right now, simply go back to the first sandwich section (starting on page 21). No judgment here.

ANYTHING SALAD SANDWICH

Tuna salad, chicken salad, egg salad, and ham salad (I'm from the South, OK?) all have something in common. They're an assemblage of things held together with mayonnaise, spices, and dreams. If you have a can of tuna—or salmon!—you're halfway to an easy, excellent sand-wich. Ditto if you have some leftover chicken or ham, or a cooked rotisserie chicken from the grocery store. If you don't eat meat, try eggs or chickpeas (this is a great use for those store-bought cooked eggs). Basically, you take your protein, dump it in a bowl, and cut or mash it into roughly bite-size pieces. Add a tablespoon or 2 of mayon-naise (or just a medium-size glob), a squirt or so of mustard, salt, and pepper, and mix it up. Add more mayo if you want it to be creamier, or a glug of olive oil. You can enhance it further if you have some other things kicking around your cupboard. A teaspoon of soy sauce is a great flavor contrast. A squeeze of lemon juice is excellent. Throwing in a little bit of something spicy, like hot sauce, harissa paste, or red pepper flakes, is also great. I like capers, celery, or cucumbers in mine for a little crunch and freshness in there. Play around with spices here, too—you never know what could be a hit. At best you now have a Secret Family Recipe you can bring to every potluck; at the very worst you've wasted some eggs.

TUNA AND ARTICHOKE HEARTS

My brilliant former colleague Emma Laperruque, author of the excel-lent cookbook *Big Little Recipes*, introduced me to this simple, super flavorful, no-mayo-involved tuna salad. Take a jar of marinated arti-choke hearts and a can of tuna. Cut up the artichoke hearts, either on a chopping board or by using kitchen shears to snip them in the jar, just until they're in bite-size pieces. Combine the drained can of tuna in a bowl with the artichokes (just the artichokes, not the marinade they're jarred in—save that, you'll need it!). Mash them together with a fork, slowly adding in the artichoke marinade until the tuna salad gets to the consistency you like. Salt and pepper it, then put it on a slice of bread. This is particularly lovely with a slice of swiss cheese or cheddar melted on it (Emma's preference), but I really like it as it is in a sandwich.

ROASTED VEGETABLES, GOAT CHEESE, AND BALSAMIC

If you recently made a sheet pan meal (page 135) and you still have roasted vegetables kicking around, you are moments from a sandwich. Heat the vegetables in the microwave if you want them warm, or use them right out of the fridge—both are good. Pile them onto toasted bread slathered with goat cheese. If you don't have goat cheese, hummus, pesto, or cream cheese also work. Drizzle the vegetables with balsamic vinegar and give them a round of black pepper.

You will basically never regret roasting a big pile of vegetables when you have the energy, by the way. In addition to this sandwich, if you have roasted vegetables you also have a lot of the fixings for soup (page 119), quesadillas (page 65), or just a bowl of vegetables maybe with an egg on top.

BLTS, BLATS, AND BECS

There's a reason that bacon was an internet obsession in the aughts. It's salty and umami, crispy and meaty, and it can really pull an entire meal together. (Brussels sprouts are delicious; brussels sprouts with bacon are a $17 appetizer at a small plates restaurant.) And you don't even need to eat pork to participate in the delights of bacon. Thanks to innovations in the plant-based-meat world, there are many bacon substitutes that offer similar levels of crispiness and saltiness. My favorite is seitan bacon, which I use in my house to make my vegetarian husband veggie BLTs. Tempeh bacon doesn't have the same texture as the meat kind but has a wonderful umami flavor of its own. There are also soy-based bacon strips that crisp up like the real thing. (Just don't attempt to grill them, like I did once, or they might catch on fire and result in you having to stomp frantically on a strip of fake meat to put out the flames. Learn from my mistakes.)

Regardless, if you have the energy to cook, bacon is a good use of that energy, because it can be the only thing you cook for a sandwich and that sandwich will be spectacular. After a certain number of grease-related injuries, I don't bother with cooking bacon in a skillet anymore. For a couple strips of bacon, you can just use the microwave (see page 102)! For larger batches of bacon, the method I prefer is putting the bacon on a sheet pan in a cold oven, then turning the temperature up to 400°F. Check it after 15 minutes to determine the level of crispiness—it might need another 5 or 10 minutes. Pull it out while it looks a little less crispy than you'd like. It'll crisp up once it comes out of the heat.

Once you have bacon (or fake-on), then you can make a BLT. It's particularly delicious when tomatoes are at their peak, but let's be real, it hits the other ten months of the year as well. Throw some avocado in the mix and you've got a BLAT. That's a meal. Beautiful. Easy. Done.

If you want to take things in a more breakfast direction, you can fry a quick egg, plop that on bread with bacon, and add a slice of American cheese for an easy BEC. Or if you don't have any of those ingredients, or making the bacon was all the energy you have today, thanks, then you don't have to bother with that. Butter some bread (or toast, if you have the willpower), sprinkle some pepper over it, layer some bacon on top, and then add another slice of bread. Bacon sandwich.

Quesadilla That Thang

If you have tortillas and some kind of cheese you have the makings of a quesadilla. Shredded cheese is ideal, but sliced will also work (and as we know, the sliced stuff melts like a dream). If you just have bricks of cheese then you'll want to shred them before using, but you can chip bits off with a knife if you don't want to use a grater, and, bonus, it might make you feel better to chip bits off something with a knife. This is a great place for cheddar, pepper jack, mozzarella, or American cheese. Sprinkle a thin layer of cheese evenly on top of one small tortilla or half a big one in a frying pan, or the closest thing you have. (If you have tortillas on hand, either is good, but if you're currently at the store shopping for quesadilla fixings, I'll note that big folded quesadillas are a little easier to flip.) The thin layer isn't because I'm cheese-phobic, I promise—it's so that it has a chance to melt. Add your chosen filling and another very thin layer of cheese, and heat on medium-high until the cheese is a little melty. Then pop on another small tortilla if you're doing that, or fold the other half of the big tortilla over. Carefully flip to warm the other side, and you're done.

You can also cook a quesadilla in the oven, rather than in a pan (which, bonus, allows you to cook multiple quesadillas at once). Stuff your tortilla (or tortillas) with cheese and your preferred filling, then slide it onto a greased sheet pan (you can just spray it with cooking spray). Put it in a 400°F degree oven. Bake it for 7 minutes, and then flip it and bake for another 3 to 5 minutes, until it looks brown and crispy.

A plain tortilla with cheese and a sprinkle of red pepper flakes inside, folded and griddled on both sides, is a perfect snack. I like to dollop mine with sour cream and salsa if I have them. You can also add easy quesadilla fillings to yours, like:

- Brie and apple slices
- Spinach, bacon, and cheddar
- Broccoli and cheddar
- Shredded zucchini and monterey jack
- Drained black beans, pickled jalapeño slices, and shredded Mexican cheese
- Cooked sweet potato chunks, refried beans, and cheddar
- Tomato slices, basil, and mozzarella
- Rotisserie chicken, avocado, and swiss cheese
- Brie and dried cranberries
- Chocolate and marshmallow (a dessert quesadilla!)

LEFTOVERSDILLA

Where quesadillas really shine is in their ability to transform leftovers. You can stuff a quesadilla with so many of the awkward little dribs and drabs hanging out in your fridge. I love a leftover chicken tandoori quesadilla, for example. If you have leftover bits of cooked chicken, fish, or beef, you can easily cut them up into bite-size pieces and tuck them into the quesadilla. Same thing with vegetables. Vegetables won't really have a chance to cook in the time that it takes for the cheese to melt and the tortilla to crisp up, which is why this is brilliant for leftovers—they're already cooked. I probably don't need to tell you that canned beans (also already cooked) are great in quesadillas, but have you considered just tossing some of that bean salad you made on page 18 in here? The main thing to remember is to make sure that anything you're using in the quesadilla is dry, or dry-ish. That's because extra liquid in the middle of the quesadilla will cause the tortilla to steam rather than crisp up. (It'll still be perfectly edible that way, though.) If you have vegetables or meat in a sauce, pat them dry of the sauce as best you can before you add it to the tortilla and cheese. If you want, you can add a handful of cheese to the pan before you add the tortilla so that it melts and browns *on* the quesadilla as well as inside it. That's called a *frico* or, in my house, a "freaky freaky frico," with apologies to the nation of Italy.

When I Dip You Dip We Dip

If you don't have the strength to assemble anything into a formal sandwich, toast, or quesadilla, or what you have on hand is more in the chips-and-crackers arena than the bread-tortilla arena, all is not lost. In fact, that guy from *Only Murders in the Building* is maybe on to something. You can easily assemble yourself a meal out of dips. I do it fairly often. My husband and I call it the Super Bowl after the American holiday most associated with eating a bunch of dips for a meal. We'll look at each other and ask, "Is it the Super Bowl today?" and if so, we'll either make an assembly of whatever we have in our pantry, or I'll do the work to make one really good but time-intensive dip—a caramelized onion and sour cream one, or a spinach and artichoke number—and then we'll sit down and eat it as a meal. No football is required. Dip for dinner is a sacred national right for all Americans.

Even if you don't have the strength to caramelize onions or layer beans you can accomplish dip for dinner. How? Well, first expand what counts in your mind as a dip, and what counts as a chip.

THINGS YOU CAN USE TO DIP

Obviously, chips are chips. But are other things also chips? Technically, perhaps no, but in the context of chips and dip, perhaps yes. Try dunking the following:

- Chips (duh)
- Tater tots, cooked from frozen
- Potato wedges
- Baby carrots
- Celery sticks
- Broccoli florets
- Sugar snap peas
- Crackers
- Robust lettuces, like romaine stems or iceberg cups
- Cheese cups
- Toast, cut into triangles
- Pita
- Flatbread, cooked from frozen

DIPS

It's not news to you, I'm sure, that salsa and guacamole are dips. But then so are hummus, ranch dressing, green goddess dressing, and pesto, and I'd count leftover chicken or tuna salad as dips too. Dig around your pantry and see what you have in there. There are some simple, easy dips you can whip up with two or three ingredients you might already have on hand.

Easy queso: Combine equal amounts of salsa and dice-size chunks of American cheese or Velveeta. Microwave for 30 seconds, then stir. Repeat until it has collapsed into a gooey, cheesy mass.

Easy chili dip: Mash together one can of chili, one block of cream cheese (or container of sour cream if that's what you have), and a solid handful (½ cup) of any shredded cheese you have on hand. Microwave for a minute, and mash again. Microwave for another 30 seconds, and see what the consistency is. Does it look like a dip? Great. You're done. Not yet? Keep microwaving for 30-second increments until the cheese is melted and it looks like a coherent mass, rather than three separate components.

Blue cheese, sour cream, and lemon: Mush up blue cheese chunks or a block of blue cheese—about ¼ pound of it, if you're measuring. Then add to a standard size container of sour cream (about 8 ounces) and mix it up. Add a squirt of lemon juice if you have it.

Salmon dip: If you have a can of salmon knocking around your pantry, then you are extremely close to having salmon dip. This also works with leftover smoked salmon, if you happen to have that. Drain the can of salmon, and mash it up with the contents of a container of sour cream. Salt and pepper liberally. If you have dill, dried or fresh, add it. If not, don't. A squeeze of lemon wouldn't go awry if you have that, too, but it's not make or break.

Sort-of raita: If you have plain yogurt or sour cream and a cucumber, you're close to a kind of dirtbag version of raita I like to make. Cut the cucumber into large-ish chunks, and put them into a food processor or blender along with a cup of yogurt or sour cream. Pulse until it becomes a consistent texture. If it doesn't seem to be coming together, add a teaspoon or so of water and pulse again. Keep doing that until you have a dip. If you don't want to use a blender, you can grate the cucumber or smash it into tiny bits, and that'll work too.

Sort-of olive tapenade: Do you have olives? Do you have anchovies? Then you have a riff on olive tapenade, one that's umami and briney and deeply savory. Make sure that your olives are pitted—that's important to prevent unpleasant tooth-cracking incidents. I usually use canned pitted black olives, or sometimes sliced olives, depending on what's around. Then combine them in a blender or food processor with a can of anchovies and a squeeze of lemon juice, if you have that around. Smear on toast or crackers.

Easy esquites: I love the Mexican corn dish elote and its cousin esquites so much—they manage to be sweet and tangy and creamy and zesty all at once. Esquites isn't technically a dip, but this pared-down version kind of works as one. Basically, you thaw a cup of frozen corn and mix it in a bowl with a tablespoon or 2 of mayonnaise, a dash of Tajín or chili powder (or more, depending on how hot you like it), a squeeze of lime juice, and a handful of crumbled cotija cheese (or feta if you can't find cotija). Stir it around so all the ingredients are incorporated, and add more chili, lime, mayo, or salt to taste, though go easy on the salt because the cheese is also pretty salty.

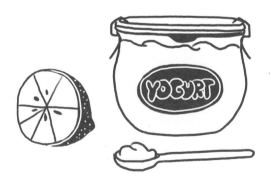

Do Exactly This: The Easiest Dip I Know

This dip can easily be supplemented by all manner of spices and spice mixes should you wish, such as everything bagel seasoning, taco seasoning, or Italian seasoning. But it's great as is—I always make it when people are coming over at the last minute, and it's always totally gone within half an hour. Labneh works instead of the yogurt or sour cream, if you happen to have that instead. Feel free to add more lemon juice, too.

Ingredients

- 1 cup *yogurt* or *sour cream*
- 1 teaspoon *garlic powder*
- 2 tablespoons *lemon juice* (or one fresh lemon, squeezed)
- *Salt and pepper*
- 2 tablespoons *olive oil*

1. Grab a medium-size bowl. Add the yogurt, garlic powder, and lemon juice, and stir together.
2. Salt and pepper the mixture aggressively—at least 2 big pinches of salt, and 3 extra shakes (or cranks of a pepper grinder) past your usual peppering instincts. Stir together. Taste—if it has picked up a pleasing savoriness, you're there. If it still mostly tastes like yogurt, add more salt and pepper to taste.
3. Swirl olive oil over the top. You've got dip.

Cowboy Caviar, the Dip That Is Also a Meal

O f all the dips that I can argue count as a full, actual meal, cowboy caviar is the most convincing. If you've never encountered it before, essentially cowboy caviar is just a bean salad held together with a sharp vinaigrette and eaten with chips. Could it count as a salad? Sure. Does eating it with chips make it feel more festive? It does, at least to me.

What goes into cowboy caviar? Basically, you grab a big bowl and add to it black-eyed peas and black beans, both drained and from a can. Then add chopped-up green or red onion, corn (thawed frozen corn is the simplest and best option), a handful of cilantro, and diced tomatoes (fresh or from a can). Toss it all together with a good amount of salt and pepper, lime juice, and a tablespoon or 2 of red wine vinegar. You can add chopped avocado or feta if you want, and you can substitute whatever other beans you have knocking around. The amounts don't really matter very much here—you can kind of just throw it all in the bowl and keep adding, mixing, and tasting until you get to a loose concoction that you like. The lawlessness is part of the charm.

Canapé and Willapé

I am a firm believer that a certain number of snacks, combined, can turn into a meal, sort of the way a certain number of children with rings can summon Captain Planet. But the trick is that the snacks need to be hearty enough that an hour later you aren't hungry again. (The ultimate indignity: managing to feed your stupid body *and then still needing to feed it!* It's bad enough that you have to do it again tomorrow.)

Cheese and crackers, as we've discussed, can definitely do the trick, as can a combination of toddler-level snacks—say, apple slices with peanut butter, a string cheese, and some carrot sticks. But as anyone who has tried to use a fancy work event as a free substitute for dinner knows, you can also collect enough party snacks to make a meal. A collection of canapés (group noun: desperation) can serve as dinner or lunch.

What's the difference between canapés and hors d'oeuvres, you ask? Canapés are always served cold, which makes them even easier to assemble into a meal than their cooked counterparts. They're basically just French finger foods that you don't need to worry about heating.

CANAPÉ BASICS (CANAPÉSICS?)

The basic formula for a canapé is base + spread + garnish. That's really it. You can be as fancy with that as you want. A classic example is a blini + crème fraîche + caviar. But I don't know about you, caviar isn't something that's usually knocking around my fridge when I'm feeling exhausted and burned out, due to my not being a Russian oligarch. Here are some more achievable combinations:

- Cracker + cream cheese + smoked salmon
- Cracker + slice of mozzarella + slice of tomato + drizzle of balsamic vinegar
- Slice of cucumber + feta + sun-dried tomato
- Baguette slice + brie + dried cranberries
- Baguette slice + goat cheese + pesto
- Cracker + cream cheese + avocado
- Cracker + hummus + cucumber

Basically, anything that sounds like a great little open-faced sandwich would probably be a good canapé. There are no hard rules, but the spread helps anchor the other things to your base; otherwise, you'll have to deal with the dread forces of gravity potentially upending the things on top of your cracker or cucumber slice (perhaps especially your cucumber slice, because they're slippery).

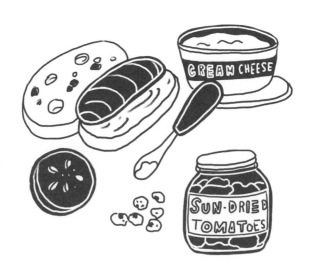

Roll Your Own Canapés

Are you ready to feast on some small bites but stuck for ideas? Roll a die to find an element from each category. Then turn those components into a snack and turn that snack into a meal.

BASES

1. Water crackers
2. Triscuits or other shredded wheat crackers
3. Rice crackers or mini rice cakes
4. Sliced cucumber
5. Sliced baguette
6. Pita chip

SPREADS

1. Hummus
2. Boursin
3. Cream cheese
4. Feta or goat cheese
5. Mashed avocado
6. Butter

GARNISHES

1. Pesto or grab-bag green sauce (page 115)
2. Smoked or tinned fish
3. Sliced black olive
4. Sliced radish
5. Prosciutto (or other sliced meat)
6. Chili crisp (or hot sauce, pepper jelly, or harissa)

Party for One

If you like the idea of a meal made of little bites of things but you'd rather have a hot meal, then we turn to hors d'oeuvres, which, again, just means "finger foods" in French. There are a whole bunch of recipes out there for delicious fiddly little bites of things, but when I'm too tired to cook, there is a zero percent chance of me dealing with sheets of puff pastry. I am also not going to make meatballs from scratch. But if the meatballs require only heating from my freezer? Yeah, I'm into that.

Luckily, the freezer section of every grocery store is simply packed with finger foods that require nothing but a quick trip through the oven to become a loose, anarchic dinner. My favorites are tiny spanakopita cups, pigs in a blanket, mini quiches, bite-size samosas, and, yes, I do consider Bagel Bites to be an hors d'oeuvre. Stocking some boxes of finger foods in your freezer isn't just good for emergency hosting, it's great for a last-minute dinner that feels kind of festive. If you have an air fryer, this is a great time to use it—getting frozen foods crispy is basically what that bad boy does. If you don't, then a toaster oven or actual oven also works great.

Do Exactly This: Three-Ingredient Mushroom Bites

There's no shame in the game of eating heated-up frozen premade pigs in a blanket for dinner. But there are also occasions when you might want to assemble something low-effort from scratch. For those times, I recommend these easy, delicious mushroom bites, involving three ingredients, two of which are cheese. They're adapted from a go-to recipe from my friend

Rachel Apatoff, a pastry enthusiast, brilliant costume designer, and the kind of person who was actually making and serving finger foods at college parties while the rest of us brought over a six-pack of warm Modelo or a suspicious-looking bottle of "infused" vodka. I have made these mushrooms for parties, sure, but I have also eaten the entire tray by myself as a meal.

Ingredients

- *8 ounces (1 container) button or cremini mushrooms*
- *1 package garlic and fine herbs Boursin*
  - *If you can't find that, another flavor of Boursin*
  - *If you can't find Boursin, a savory flavored cream cheese, like scallion cream cheese*
- *¼ cup (4 heaping spoonfuls) grated parmesan or pecorino*

1. Heat your oven to 350°F. Find a baking sheet. Wash the mushrooms, and then remove the stems from them so you just have the bowl-like tops. We're not doing anything with the stems here, so you can save them for a different application or just compost them. (This does not count as chopping anything because the stems pop right out—it's fun.)

2. Take a spoon and fill a mushroom top with a small dollop of Boursin. The amount will differ based on the size of the mushroom cap, but aim to completely fill the spot where the stem was. Then put the mushroom cheese side up on the baking sheet. Repeat with all the mushrooms, lining them up on the baking sheet. Don't worry about overcrowd-

ing—we're not trying to get them crispy here, just melty. Sprinkle parmesan or pecorino on top of each of the cheese-filled mushrooms.

3. Pop the sheet pan of mushrooms into the hot oven. Bake for 8 to 10 minutes, until you see a little pool of water form under the mushrooms (we want them to release some of their liquid, but not cook so long that they turn into limp brown blobs). Let them cool a little so the melted cheese doesn't scald your mouth, but otherwise you can eat these right off the baking sheet. Party!

Nachos Are a State of Mind

In the early 2010s, when I was in grad school and in need of a distraction, I started a short-lived blog called *The Nacho Project* dedicated to the glory of nachos. Not only are nachos fun to eat and often extremely tasty, they're also an endlessly versatile canvas for fun food experiments. I made Indian-inspired nachos with saag paneer and garlic pickle, and pot pie nachos with pieces of puff pastry as the chips and a mushroom gravy as the cheese sauce. I made waffle nachos (layering toaster waffles with various nacho ingredients) *and* nacho waffles (putting cheese and jalapeños in waffle batter and then eating the waffles layered with salsa and sour cream). You can do so many things with nachos. I believe they are one of the most perfect foods, particularly when you aren't up for doing a lot of cooking but assembling something feels just fine. (I also believe nachos are a kind of salad—if pasta salad and potato salad exist, why don't nachos count, huh?—but I've run into trouble with the salad pedants before with this anarcho-salad hot take.) In conclusion, I love and admire nachos, and when I can't figure out what else to eat, they're always a good place to turn.

You don't have to use any of those experimental flavors to appreciate a home nacho dinner (or lunch). A good old-fashioned sheet pan full of nachos makes for a meal that can clean out the fridge, convey some basic nutrients, and be eaten with your hand on the couch, if that's your vibe. It's also incredibly easy to scale up or down a nacho meal. If you need to feed a larger group, just add more sheet pans to the mix. If you're looking for a single-serve portion of nachos, you don't have to use the whole sheet pan. (You can also make nachos for one in the toaster oven, on the toaster oven pan.)

What are the principles of nachos? Simple. You're looking for layers of toppings, all supported by an undergirding of chips that will allow you to scoop up delicious things and eat them. A good sturdy tortilla chip is ideal, but we just don't live in an ideal world, so use whatever's in reach—and yes, Doritos work.

MAKE TWO CATEGORIES OF INGREDIENTS: HOT AND COLD

Dig around in the fridge and see what you have that would be good on nachos, and divide it into two piles: stuff you want to make hot, and stuff you want to keep cold. Good nachos are a mixture of both— warm melty cheese and cool dollops of sour cream, hot pockets of beans and crunchy slices of radishes.

The most crucial warm ingredient, and indeed the most crucial element of nachos, is the cheese. And yes, American cheese is great here—melting down Velveeta into a sauce and dribbling it over nachos is incredible. But basically, any shredded cheese will work, like cheddar, pepper jack, or monterey jack. (If you don't eat dairy, there are many really great vegan cheese options for pouring over nachos too—just make sure they have good reviews for meltiness.) You can use the grated parmesan that you bought for pasta, as long as it's the real kind and not the stuff in a shaker. Leave fancier aged goudas and whatnot for eating with crackers. You *can* use other, less meltable cheeses, but they require more work, and I dream of nachos, I do not dream of labor.

Other great ingredients to add to the warm pile: canned black or refried beans, shredded rotisserie chicken, already-cooked vegetables, crumbled seitan or soy chorizo, cooked ground meat (real or faux). Things you want to keep cold and layer on later include cilantro, radishes, sour cream, green onion, salsa (it can go either way, but I leave salsa for after the oven), pickled jalapeño rings, pickled or raw sliced red onion, guacamole or diced avocado, canned sliced black olives, crema, and lime juice.

LINE A SHEET PAN WITH FOIL AND HEAT THE OVEN TO 400°F

I usually don't advocate for covering sheet pans in foil, but in this case I make an exception because you're melting cheese, and scrubbing melted cheese off a sheet pan is one of my least favorite activities. If you want to skip the foil, by all means do. Then turn your oven on to 400°F and wait for it to heat up while you do nacho assembly.

LAYER, LAYER, LAYER

Start with a good layer of chips scattered over your sheet pan. Then, before adding other ingredients, sprinkle a serious handful of shredded cheese onto the chips. The chips are the bricks and the cheese is the mortar, and this is why I am not an architect. Once you have chips and cheese down, then go nuts with whatever other things you want on your nachos. Dollop on beans, scatter your meats, and attempt to distribute them reasonably evenly. After that you could add another layer of chips, depending on how chip-heavy you like your nachos, but I usually just add another hearty sprinkling of cheese over all the ingredients. Then slide the sheet pan into the oven. Bake for 10 to 15 minutes, until all the cheese is melted and the ingredients are warmed through.

INTEGRATE THE COLD INGREDIENTS

Once the nachos are heated through, take them out of the oven and scatter on all your cold ingredients, dolloping however you please. At this point the main concern is time—the longer the chips sit under your layers of toppings, the more likely they are to get soggy. Sogginess is the opposite of godliness, nachos-wise, so the solution is simply to eat them without delay, something I trust you can do. You can serve and eat them right off the sheet pan if you like, and not bother with transferring them to a plate, but the sheet pan will be hot so be careful not to burn yourself. You can also just scoot the foil that the nachos are on onto another serving plate or sheet pan, and eat them from there, particularly if kids are eating and you're worried about eager little hands getting scorched.

You Go, Gurt

On the sitcom *Brooklyn 99*, there is a running joke that a sergeant named Terry Jeffords, portrayed by the extremely talented and ripped

Terry Crews, is obsessed with yogurt. He is constantly eating yogurt, seemingly for every meal, and I know that it's just a sitcom-y affectation, but I hard relate. Yogurt is incredible. You can add salt, pepper, and lemon juice, and voilà: a dip (see page 71). If you throw some spices, olive oil, and vinegar into it, it becomes a marinade. If you stir dill, garlic, and parsley in there you get something like yogurt ranch dressing, incredible for dressing up lackluster proteins or shoveling into your mouth with baby carrots or shards of bell pepper. But perhaps more importantly for when you're feeling too overwhelmed to do anything but spoon delicious goo into your face, yogurt is a terrific base for a light, filling meal. You can stir fruit into it and, wow, a parfait. Do you have a little jam? Maybe a sprinkling of nuts? A luscious, easy breakfast treat. Or bulk it up with something crunchy and take it savory for lunch or, sure, why not, dinner.

There's an entire spectrum of yogurts out there, from the fruit-on-the-bottom cups to the thicker, tangy Greek-style guys to heavy, mild Icelandic skyr. If you're dairy-averse, there are also a number of delicious coconut yogurts I have sometimes accidentally purchased and not regretted. All of them have their merits. Personally, I am a devotee of full-fat plain Greek yogurt, and it is rare that I don't have a giant tub of it in my fridge. Full-fat dairy is perhaps the smallest hill I'm willing to die on. Until I was in my mid-twenties I lived by the law of reduced-fat dairy, because I am a child of the '90s and that is what I was taught. It was only after accidentally using whole milk in an iced coffee that I discovered a fundamental truth: full-fat dairy tastes better, *and* it's more satisfying. Life is short! Full fat only means like 5 percent fat, not 100 percent fat! Only you know what makes sense for your life and dietary requirements, but for real, try full-fat yogurt sometime if you haven't.

ASSEMBLE! THAT! YOGURT!

No matter your preferred fat content or thickness of yogurt, you can easily turn regular, plain yogurt into a meal thanks to our friend toppings. Like oatmeal, yogurt dishes tend to go sweet—like the (deservedly) omnipresent yogurt, granola, and fruit parfait—and yogurt is delicious that way. But the truth is that you can easily take things in a savory direction, too. Greek yogurt is not that far off from cream cheese, for example—you can layer it on toast with salt and pepper and some slices of avocado, and voilà, a meal. Lox and yogurt: why not? It's also good with salt and pepper under a crispy egg, or in a bowl topped with a drizzle of olive oil, some crispy chickpeas, and a handful of cherry tomatoes.

There aren't any rules when making a yogurt meal. But if you're a yogurt-mixing beginner still figuring out what you like, I recommend adding two things: an extra flavor ingredient, whether sweet or savory, and something that provides textural contrast. If you don't like texture in your yogurt, I get it—I am married to a person who loves nothing more than a mush—but for me, I like there to be something that stands out from the yogurt's creaminess. It can be chewy, crispy, or crunchy: dry cereal, sunflower seeds, wheat germ, crumbled nori, or dried berries or fruit (which can complement either sweet or savory yogurt, and is a shelf-stable way to achieve the classic fruit-and-yogurt combo). This is another great place to break out your spices—cinnamon, cardamom, and ginger go great with sweet yogurt applications. For a savory direction, try stirring in a little bit of chili powder or cumin, or a pinch of dried herbs. (For maximum success I suggest buying plain yogurt, rather than the kind that has fruit or some other flavor like vanilla. Those are great, too, but they limit your flavor options somewhat, or at least lock you into a sweeter direction.)

Try some of these topping combos to turn your yogurt into a meal—
or mix and match the ones that sound good to you.

Sweet toppings

- Peanut butter + granola
- Dollop of jam + handful of chopped nuts
- Swirl of lemon curd + crumbled graham crackers
- Sliced bananas + dried coconut flakes
- Cinnamon + chopped-up apples
- Dried cranberries + chocolate chips
- Berries + chia seeds
- Drizzle of tahini + cut-up dried figs
- Drizzle of honey + sunflower seeds

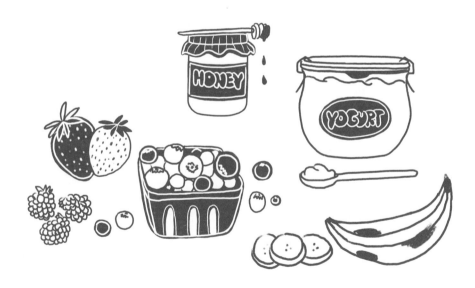

Savory toppings

- Olive oil + lemon juice + arugula
- Chili crisp
- Everything bagel seasoning
- Olive oil + sliced radishes
- Grated garlic + cut-up cucumber
- Salt + pepper + fried egg
- Avocado + crumbled nori
- Crispy chickpeas + za'atar
- Pesto + sun-dried tomatoes
- Leftover roasted vegetables + drizzle of balsamic vinegar
- Cut-up cherry tomatoes + crumbled corn chips

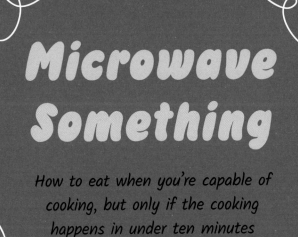

Microwave Something

How to eat when you're capable of cooking, but only if the cooking happens in under ten minutes and you mainly push a button

n this, the age of the air fryer and the Instant Pot, the original convenience device gets a bad rap. But the microwave is an absolutely glorious thing, particularly when you want to have a meal quickly. It's basically a very small steam oven, which makes it ideal for quickly cooking or reheating all kinds of things. Yes, of course, there's popcorn, but you can also cook eggs, bacon, vegetables, and rice in the microwave. It's not the right tool for when you want to get food crispy, as anyone who has attempted to reheat some french fries in the microwave can tell you, but otherwise, it's incredible for putting together a meal with a minimum of dirty dishes and fuss. It's also great when, say, you can't deal with your oven because it's too hot outside, or all your pots and pans are in an unmanageable pile in the sink. You're cooking, but the cooking happens in under ten minutes and requires very little effort. That's the dream!

Popcorn: A Manifesto

Popcorn for dinner is a classic of the genre. It's fun, it has the feeling of a semispecial occasion, and it means that you can completely ignore the dishes for a minute. It doesn't require much more than a microwave (or, if you just have the kernels, a microwave and a paper bag). And then you can top it with all kinds of things that make it into more of a meal.

What if you don't have microwave popcorn, just popcorn kernels? No problem. You can always pop popcorn the old-fashioned way, by putting it into a giant pot with a slick of oil at the bottom and heating it on the stove until that whole pot fills with delicious, fluffy kernels. But if you, like me, want popcorn for dinner or a snack specifically because you are trying not to mess with stoves and pots, don't worry. Any popcorn can be microwave popcorn. Here's how.

MAKE ANY POPCORN INTO MICROWAVE POPCORN

Grab your unpopped kernels and a paper bag. The kind that you pack a lunch in is ideal. Mix ½ cup of popcorn kernels (you *do* have to measure this properly, sorry; popcorn kernels expand enormously and can easily overwhelm their container, so you don't want to just vibe it out) with a teaspoon of oil (or a good glug if you don't feel like measuring), and pour them into the paper bag. Fold the top of the bag over 3 times, so it has a good seal. Microwave on high for 3 minutes, listening to hear the corn popping. When it slows to a pop every couple of seconds, pull it out. Open the bag, being careful of the wall of popcorn steam that inevitably accompanies bagged popcorn. Top it with anything you want. Voilà, popcorn.

Don't have a paper bag? Still not a problem. Put ½ cup of unpopped kernels, again lightly coated in oil, in a microwavable glass bowl. Use one that feels slightly too big—trust me, it's better than having one that's too small and making an accidental popcorn flood. Cover the bowl with a plate. Microwave on high for 3 to 5 minutes, listening for the popping to slow down. Use oven mitts to take the bowl out of the microwave and remove the plate. Behold, popcorn.

BEYOND PLAIN POPCORN

Popcorn toppings are a personal thing, and I get that. My in-laws sometimes eat olives on theirs. It's not for me but I respect the innovation. Olive oil or melted butter and salt are great. If you love movie theater style popcorn, might I suggest ordering some Flavacol? It's the butter-flavored seasoning that gets tossed onto popcorn at the movies (not the fake butter topping, that's a different thing). You can buy it on Amazon or other places online, and it comes in what looks like a giant milk carton. A teaspoon sprinkled onto your popcorn will give you that theater-style *oomph*—and that carton will outlive us all, so if you have the shelf space, you have popcorn toppings in perpetuity. Here are a few other ideas for giving your popcorn a little extra zip, or to bulk it up into more of a meal-feeling item rather than a snack one. For dry seasonings, spray or drizzle a small amount of oil to coat the popcorn kernels before adding the powdered seasoning—it'll help it stick to the kernels better.

Old faithfuls

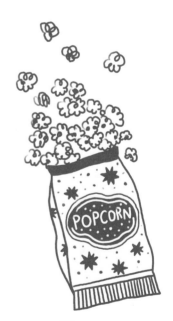

- Butter and salt
- Black pepper and parmesan
- Dried oregano or Italian seasoning
- Nutritional yeast

Fun flavors

- Furikake
- Soy sauce and sugar
- Cajun seasoning
- Hot sauce

- Powdered ranch dressing
- Taco mix
- Curry powder
- Tomato powder

It's a meal now

- Prosciutto and slivered pecorino
- Diced avocado and sun-dried tomatoes
- Trail mix
- Arugula and capers

Oatmeal Best Meal

I am of Irish extraction—my mother grew up in Athlone, the center part of the country that no tourist has ever heard of. As a result, my family is incredibly serious about oatmeal or, as we call it, porridge. My family mail-orders Flahavan's oatmeal, and absolutely swears by it, but unless you, too, have an auntie who travels with her own specific porridge oats, you are allowed to just grab whatever's around.

OATMEAL TAXONOMY

If you look in the cereal aisle of the grocery store, there are generally three kinds of oats: steel-cut, rolled (or "old-fashioned"), and quick-cooking. The only real reason these distinctions are important is that they have different cooking times, so pay attention to the label of the container when preparing oatmeal. Steel-cut oats take the longest to cook, then rolled oats, and then—no points for guessing—quick-cooking. No matter what kind you have, oats stay good on the shelf for simply ever and oatmeal is one of the easiest things to make on the planet. The hardest preparation, which is still easy, is to put it in a pot with water or milk and simmer it until the oats lose their bite and turn into a pleasing mush. (The package will tell you how much liquid to use.) The easiest is to microwave it (best for quick or rolled oats) or leave it in a slow cooker overnight (better for the steel-cut guys). That's gruel, baby.

SWEET OATMEAL

Oats are great as a base for a meal because you can throw a lot of things at them. Oatmeal's an accommodating mush that way. There's a tendency to lean sweet when it comes to oats—a dab of honey, some brown sugar, and a shake of cinnamon (or, even better, apple pie spice or pumpkin spice), and you're on your way. Maple syrup or molasses is good in them, as is a pile of whatever berries you have around (you can use frozen—the hot oatmeal will unfreeze them), or a cut-up banana. You can swirl in a spoonful of Nutella, or peanut butter and jam for an oat-y take on the classic sandwich. Dried fruits, like raisins, cranberries, apricots, or prunes, also play really well in oatmeal, as does shredded coconut. Chopped nuts add a nice little bit of crunch to the endeavor. Chocolate chips or even chopped-up candy bars will work, or mini marshmallows. Dig around your pantry—I bet you have something that could work in a classic bowl of sweet oatmeal.

SAVORY OATMEAL

But where things *really* get going, for me, is when you steer oatmeal in a savory direction. Just make sure that your oats don't have any added sugar—some quick oats have it included in the packet. You can cook the oatmeal in broth instead of water, or add bouillon or the flavor packet from a pack of ramen for extra zazz, or add some ginger and garlic to the cooking water.

If that's too much to deal with, fret not. Though my mother is Irish, I grew up in Alabama, and so I learned that you can treat oatmeal like grits. Add a pinch of salt and a pat of butter, or stir in a handful of shredded cheese. A fried, scrambled, or soft-boiled egg on top with a lot of black pepper ground over it is amazing, as is a drizzle of chili oil, hot sauce, or chili crisp. You can throw shredded chicken or cooked shrimp over the bowl, or chunks of avocado and a couple scoops of salsa. You can also just swirl in a spice mixture, like garam masala or berbere. Brown butter and capers are pretty great, too, for a kind of oatmeal piccata. Oats are a perfect blank canvas for weird experiments with condiments, and for leftover cooked vegetables like spinach or mushrooms, or even chunks of sweet potato or squash. Pulled pork on top with barbecue sauce? Heaven.

If this is actually *too* much freedom for you and you're having trouble choosing savory add-ins, consider: What tastes do you like? Would you like for that taste to also be hearty and filling? Great, do that. Like oatmeal the color, oatmeal the flavor is a neutral that basically goes with anything.

Hot Potato

There are killjoys out there who will tell you that a baked potato isn't good unless it's actually *baked*, you know, *in the oven*. I understand that in a perfect world, you would turn on the oven and wait the interminable 45 minutes to an hour that this requires. But you could also . . . just not do that and use the microwave instead. Microwaves are essentially steam ovens. They rule for reheating things that are liquidy, or when you don't care about food getting browned or crispy. So yes, if you absolutely need your baked potato to have a brown crispy jacket, you will have to use a toaster oven, air fryer, or, sure, an actual oven. But if you just want to be eating a potato 10 minutes from now, the microwave absolutely rules. My Irish auntie Eilish even has a handy device specifically for the microwave: a cloth pocket you tuck a potato into (she has distributed one to every member of the family). Microwave potatoes are endorsed by an actual Irish person.

BAKED POTATO BASICS

Baked potatoes are filling enough that with just a few additions they can be a whole meal, particularly when you can't deal with turning on the oven. Maybe your microwave already has a baked potato setting—mine does. All you really need to do is locate a potato (russets are best for this, but whatever works, honestly), wash it, and pierce that sucker all over with a sharp paring knife or the tines of a fork. Don't skip this part or your potato will explode. That sounds kind of cool but in practice is just a very annoying thing to have to clean out of your microwave.

Then put the potato on a plate. Microwave on high for 5 minutes, flip it over, and microwave it again for another 5 minutes. That's it. Just 10 minutes. From there you can cut the potato open and layer on the toppings. Sour cream, cheddar, chives, and bacon bits are a classic combination, but it's also a blank potato template to do whatever you want with—like oatmeal, potato is a pretty neutral flavor that can stand up to any taste you enjoy. I've put salsa and leftover taco filling on mine, and also arugula and green goddess dressing. Shredded rotisserie chicken plus Caesar dressing and some pecorino may sound weird but makes a delicious Caesar salad–adjacent potato. Black beans work incredibly well on a potato too, if you want to add in some quick vegetarian protein. Basically any cheese is also nice, thinly sliced or shredded. You can even slice open the potato, put cheese on it, and pop it back in the microwave for 30 seconds to 1 minute to melt the cheese. If you want something lower effort, treat that potato like you would popcorn. You can sprinkle on Cajun seasoning, curry powder, taco seasoning, or whatever other spice mix you have kicking around, and it'll make the potato delicious. If you have a jar of Indian curry sauce, use some of that and frozen peas to make a deconstructed samosa. Dig around in your fridge for bits of things that might taste good with a potato—hello, chili crisp—and throw them on there. And if all else fails, salt, pepper, and butter are excellent.

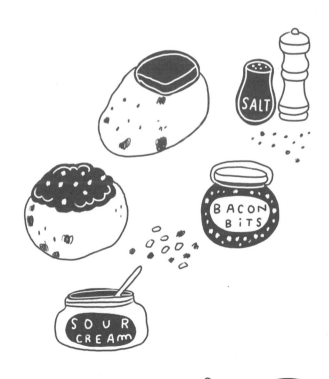

Butter Is Magic

If you're surveying the contents of your fridge for a potential meal, don't sleep on butter. Butter is one of those ingredients that can turn a pile of food into a *dish*.

You might be shocked by how much a little dollop of butter can smooth everything out and amplify flavors. When I was in culinary school, someone asked how much butter to add to a sauce and the chef shrugged and said "up to a half cup," which is an entire stick, so don't ever feel bad about liberal butter usage. Adding a little butter to a sauce or saucy dish to finish it, by the way, is a French technique called *monter au beurre*, so actually when you put butter on noodles, rice, oatmeal, or vegetables you are being a *chef*.

If you want something a little more elegant without working much harder, you can also brown the butter. This technique sounds fancy and delicate, but it's really just melting butter in a pan and cooking out the water content. Over medium-low heat, melt the butter and keep cooking it. It'll usually foam up somewhat, but then the foam will collapse. What you're looking for is the little bits in the melted butter—those are milk solids—to turn a toasty brown. That'll usually take 5 to 7 minutes, and the pan will start smelling nutty. Once it hits that point, pull the pan off the heat. (If you keep going, the butter could burn.) Then dump it on your pasta or literally anything else.

Marcella Hazan, queen of Italian cooking, has an amazingly popular sauce that's just an onion, cut in half and peeled, dumped in a pot with a 28-ounce can of whole tomatoes and a stick of butter, and simmered for 45 minutes. That's it. Another easy pasta sauce? Add a dollop of tomato sauce to melted butter. Just got a plain bowl of rice? Add soy sauce and a pat of butter. Want your cheese and crackers to taste cheesier? Spread butter on a cracker before you put cheese on it, a French trick. Butter is wonderful, and it is the keystone of so many cuisines. Add a dollop or a schmear and see if it improves your life. It just might.

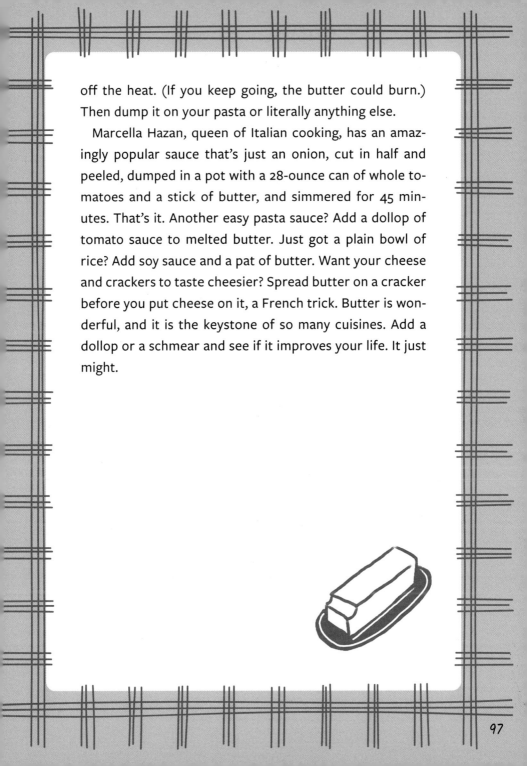

Rice in a Mug

I have an ongoing relationship with my rice cooker, an incredible machine that means that the days of making rice that is somehow simultaneously undercooked and burned are behind me. I do recommend having a rice cooker (they are often inexpensive and really do make your life easier), but you can definitely get by without one. The easiest way I know to make rice, besides the appliance literally dedicated to and created for that pursuit, is in the microwave. It also means that you can make a small amount of rice in a mug if you like the idea of having some rice but the process of filling a pot and boiling water and watching it fills you with despair. I understand! I have been there.

All you need is a microwave-safe mug or bowl, rice, water, and salt. Remember that whatever amount of dry rice you use will turn into triple that amount of cooked rice. So 1 cup of uncooked rice makes 3 cups of cooked rice, and ⅓ cup of rice turns into 1 cup of cooked rice, which is a great serving for one person.

Let's say you're making a cup of jasmine rice in a mug, because that's what I do. Add ⅓ cup of uncooked rice to a mug with a pinch of salt in there, and pour in ⅔ cup of water—in other words, fill the mug one-third of the way with rice and then top off with water. (This works for medium-grain white rice that's commonly found in giant bags in the grocery store—sushi rice, risotto rice, black rice, or brown rice have their own rules.) Then put the mug in the microwave and microwave it for 5 minutes. Take it out and stir the rice. Taste a grain. Is it soft or still pretty crunchy? If crunchy, microwave again for 2 minutes. Keep going in this fashion until the rice is to your liking. Then you have a mug of rice, and you don't even have to clean an extra dish. If you want to make more rice, use the same proportions—for instance, 1 cup of uncooked rice to 2 cups of water—but start with a proportionally longer cooking time, say 10 minutes.

Eggs Over Really Easy

If you're familiar with cooking shows or any part of the extended Anthony Bourdain universe, you know that cooking an egg perfectly is hard. It's a whole thing! In culinary school I learned that the ideal texture for a French omelet is *baveuse*—that translates to "slobbery," and was described to me as "like baby drool"—and it took the wholesale murder of eighteen eggs for me to achieve that gross-sounding but apparently desirable result.

But here's the thing: the people who decided that this is the best way to serve and consume an egg were literally French aristocrats, and I'm not really with them on their landscaping/wig/class oppression decisions, so I'm not sure why we continue to allow them to set the bar for egg preparation. Because maybe it's hard to make a perfect egg, but making an imperfect but extremely delicious egg is *easy*. You don't need to fuss over your egg for it to taste good and deliver macronutrients to your body. And wanting to eat an egg without having to do too much cooking doesn't mean you need to crack it in a glass and chug it Rocky-style. You don't even need to use a pan or an oven, which is convenient if your pan is in a pile of dirty dishes you can't possibly attend to right now. All you need is a microwave-proof container, like a mug or a Pyrex glass measuring cup. Also eggs, you do need eggs.

MICROWAVE EGG (SCRAMBLED EDITION)

Here's what you do: crack an egg or 2 into the mug and use a fork to swish it up until the yolk and white are roughly mashed together. Add some salt and pepper, and a splash of water or milk if you have it. If you feel fancy you can add some spices like cumin or garam masala, or the shake from the bottom of a bag of Doritos (that stuff is gold).

Then microwave it for 30 seconds on high. Take it out and scramble the egg. If you have some shredded cheese around, you could add it at this point, but you don't have to. Microwave again for another 30 seconds. See if the egg is set (opaque, kind of Jell-O consistency), and check that there's no unappealing loose egg white snot. If there is, throw it in for another 15 to 30 seconds. When it's done, you can dump it on an English muffin and throw a little salsa on that. You can eat it with a little toast, or scooped on some chips or crackers, or, let's be honest, wait for it to cool a little and then just eat it right out of the mug. Protein! Nutrients! Converting raw materials into a cooked meal!

MICROWAVE EGG (NOT SCRAMBLED EDITION)

If you're like "wait, I love this but I want an egg to not be scrambled," OK, I respect that! This method still works. Take your mug or dish or Pyrex measuring cup or promotional novelty bowl and grease it—butter works, or literally any edible oil would too. I don't know your life, but maybe there's a jar of coconut oil lingering in your cabinet from 2016. (Smell it to make sure it's not rancid.) Nonstick cooking spray works too. Olive oil. Canola oil. You get it.

Then crack an egg into your container. Don't stir it, but a dash of salt and pepper on that bad boy won't hurt. Soy sauce? Also great. Sprinkle it with a little bit of water. Cover it with something that can also go in the microwave—I've used a saucer and also a particularly robust coaster—and microwave for 30 seconds. Check how set it is. You'll probably want to zap it for at least another 30 seconds, depending on the age and power of your microwave. Basically, keep going in 15-second increments until the white is set and the yolk is as runny as you want it to be (anything from dark orange and custardy to light yellow and solid). Usually in my microwave it's about 1 minute for an egg over easy (the softest yolk) and 1 minute and 30 seconds for one over medium (a little bit set but still runny in the very center). That not-quite-set yolk center will be perfect for popping like the goo balloon it is. I haven't ventured into the over hard egg world too much, but you do you—if you want a fully set yolk, just keep microwaving. It won't have the crispy edges of an egg fried in a pan, but honestly, who cares. There are no egg police. Jacques Pépin is not going to break into your house and lecture you about omelets; that man is busy and has other things to deal with.

GO NUTS ON YOUR EGG

The best part of microwaved eggs is that they're also a vehicle for lots of other weird leftover scraps you might have. You can add a slice of American cheese in the final 30 seconds of cooking for it to get all melty, or mix in some cut-up leftover vegetables, or drizzle a spoonful of chili crisp on it. You can add butter or hot sauce or Golden Mountain sauce or ranch, or pretty much any other sauce you might have found lurking in your condiment treasures. You can add the egg to a bowl of grains and vegetables, or to a tortilla, or on top of some fresh-out-of-the-toaster frozen hash browns. But you absolutely don't have to do any of that, either. If all that sounds too exhausting, you just eat that egg right out of the cup you made it in. Boom—you egged.

Makin' the Bacon

If you want to turn your microwave eggs into a full microwave breakfast, what you need is microwave bacon! This method is also handy if you want bacon as a topping for your baked potato, sandwich, or salad but dealing with the grease splatters and the clean-up feels too hard. You just take out a trusty microwave-safe plate and layer it with a paper towel or two to soak up the grease. Then lay down strips of bacon on the plate so that they're not touching. Some people will tell you to adjust the power setting on the microwave to 50 percent but I have never touched the power button on my microwave and I'm not about to start now. Then nuke the bacon for 4 minutes and check it. If it's crispy enough for your liking, pull it out of the microwave now. If not, microwave for 1-minute intervals, checking after each, until it's crispy enough for you.

Emergency Cake

Cake! It's bread that has dreams, as my wise friend John once told me. But it's inconveniently difficult to make, and it requires, you know, bowls and whisks and whatnot. Also, if you make a cake or even buy a cake, you now have a whole cake to deal with, which is great if you continue to desire cake at a steady or even increasing rate, but kind of a curse if you're done after a slice and the rest of it is just hanging around going stale. Mug cakes solve both these problems because, as the name suggests, they are the size of a mug and require only a mug. The problem is that they're often tough because it's easy to overcook them, or they have streaks of flour in there because, you know, you're just mixing things in a mug and not being all that thorough (nor should you have to be).

The secret to making mug cakes that don't suck is, first, to err on the size of undercooking rather than overcooking them. And second, rather than futzing around with butter, eggs, and all the other cake trappings, what if . . . you didn't? In fact, what if you turned to an ingredient that already has heavy cream, sugar, and eggs in it—namely, ice cream? [Hold for applause.]

WHAT IF ICE CREAM, BUT IT'S CAKE

Now, some might say that if you have ice cream on hand, you already have a treat. But you know and I know that when you want cake, no other sweet thing will do. Not ice cream, not cookies, not the Halloween candy that you excavated from the back of the cupboard. This recipe will turn the dessert you are not excited about into one you are. You can also stick a candle in this if you're having a solo celebration, or if you're not and you want to be. Try that with a pint of ice cream! You can't. Well, you can, but it'll melt.

This recipe takes inspiration from a retro ice cream bread recipe, which is the kind of baking I can get down with. You can use pretty much any flavor you have on hand—I've had success with butter pecan, chocolate, vanilla, and even a fancy Earl Grey with honeycomb bits flavor I got from my favorite Philadelphia ice cream spot, Milk Jawn. The flavor in the cake is all in the ice cream, so keep that in mind when selecting a pint from your freezer. (This recipe uses ⅔ cup of ice cream, so if you have half a pint or a little less, you have enough.) You will need to have self-rising flour on hand; this is different from all-purpose flour because it already has things that help baking in it, specifically baking powder and salt. If all you have is all-purpose flour, don't worry—just add a pinch of salt and a pinch of baking powder to your flour and proceed.

You might remember that on page 14 I said there was one recipe in this book for which you can't really eyeball measurements—this is that recipe. Sorry, pals, you will need a ⅓ cup measuring cup for this! If you don't have a measuring cup but you have a set of measuring spoons, that's 5 tablespoons plus 1 teaspoon.

Do Exactly This: Two-Ingredient Mug Cake

Cakes usually contain sugar and eggs, and ice cream, conveniently, already has those things included in the mix, allowing you to swap multiple ingredients for just one. Use whatever ice cream flavor you want here, including the kind with a lot of fun little mix-ins like marshmallows or pretzel bits or chocolate fish or what have you. The extra bits provide nice little pockets of texture in the cake.

Ingredients

- ⅔ cup ice cream, any flavor
- ⅓ cup self-rising flour
  - If you don't have self-rising flour: ⅓ cup all-purpose flour, plus one pinch salt and one pinch baking powder

1. Scoop your ice cream into a mug (a small bowl will work too). Melt it by microwaving it for 30-second intervals.
2. With a fork, whisk in the self-rising flour until it's thoroughly combined (no flour streaks in there). Then microwave the mug for 1 minute.
3. Take the mug out and check the cake. Is it puffed up and looking like a baked good? Awesome, you're done. Is it still mostly liquid? Microwave for another 30 seconds.
4. Put more ice cream on top if you want, or dust with powdered sugar, or add sprinkles. Or just eat it. It's cake in a mug!

Blend Something

How to eat when a blender or food processor is accessible but chewing sounds kinda hard

Yes, I know that I sound like a small appliance evangelist from the mid-century, but I really have to say: a good blender or food processor is an incredible thing. When you don't feel like chopping things up but do feel like having some fruits and vegetables in your intake, there's nothing better than dumping a bunch of things into a blender, adding a liquid, and letting it run until it becomes, as if by magic, a smoothie. But a blender does so much more than smoothies. You can make easy vegetable soup! You can turn cans of chickpeas into hummus! You can transform all the weird wilty greens in your fridge into a zippy, clever sauce! Plus, it's a great way to whip air into something so that it becomes a different texture, like cream cheese, cottage cheese, or feta. This is why you can pry my Vitamix (bought refurbished, thanks so much) from my unwilling, smoothie-spattered hands.

Smoothie Bug-Out Bag

God, I love smoothies. They're a great breakfast for breakfast procrastinators, like myself. Smoothies are cold and refreshing, pack in nutrients, and are a good way to prevent a terrible habit of mine in which I forget to eat anything of substance until 1 p.m. and then wonder why I'm so tired and hungry. They're also a great pick-me-up for that dreaded 3 p.m. sleepy zone, and a quick way to get a bunch of fruit and vegetables in when you're feeling undernourished. They're endlessly adaptable, accommodating any dietary restriction and preference. They're a great way to use up fruit that's about to turn into slime. I have a couple every week.

It's also easy to stock your freezer and pantry with smoothie-friendly substances so you always have on hand what you need to make one. For a satisfying smoothie, you want to consider the following categories.

FROZEN FRUIT

Sure, you *could* use fresh fruit and ice for a smoothie. There's absolutely nothing wrong with that. But frozen fruit is generally more economical than its fresh cousin, and by swapping it in, you can skip the ice altogether. That means a more flavorful smoothie that's still lovely and cold. If you have too much fruit on hand from, say, an overenthusiastic visit to Costco or the farmers market, you can always put it in the freezer for later. Put cut-up fruit in ice cube trays to freeze so they don't all lump together in a giant Frankenfruit. Then you can transfer it into a zip-top bag to free up the ice cube tray, or just leave it there until you use it.

LIQUID

There's no rule that you need to use anything in smoothies aside from water. But the liquid you use in a smoothie can add flavor and more nutrients to the mix. Try milk or plant milk, kefir, orange juice, or even iced coffee—why not. Probably do not try beer, cola, or energy drinks, although I'm not going to physically stop you. Make sure that you have enough liquid to cover the rest of your smoothie ingredients by about an inch so that it's easy to blend it all together. If you don't use enough liquid, your blender will probably seize up and you'll need to mix the stuff inside around so it all gets evenly blended. It's not the end of the world, but it's kind of messy and annoying and easy to avoid by adding more of whatever liquid you want to use.

THICKENERS

The viscosity of a smoothie is personal preference, but I like mine to be fairly thick. That's a lot to do with the stuff-to-liquid ratio—the less liquid, the thicker the smoothie—but you can also add some things into the mixture that will enhance the texture of the drink. My personal favorite is a banana, especially a frozen banana, but you can also throw in a dollop or two of Greek yogurt, a couple spoonfuls of your favorite nut butter, an avocado (these freeze up great for smoothies, though the texture comes out a little suspicious for guacamole), a handful of chia seeds or rolled oats, or some cut-up zucchini.

SWEETENERS

If you like your smoothies on the sweeter side, you'll probably want to throw in something to enhance the natural sweetness of the fruits (and vegetables) in your drink. You could use straight-up granulated sugar if you want, but that can be intensely sweet, as well as ending up grainy. A liquid sweetener will make things easier. Agave syrup, maple syrup, honey, even a little bit of vanilla ice cream all work here. You can also make simple syrup if all you have is granulated white sugar. Just put ¼ cup of sugar in a heatproof vessel and pour ¼ cup of boiling water over it. Stir until the sugar dissolves, and use at will (it will keep in the fridge basically forever).

Roll Your Own Smoothie

If you're stuck on the path to a good smoothie, here's a good way to break out of the rut. Roll a die to reveal one or two frozen fruits or vegetables, a liquid, thickener, and up to two optional extras. Dump them into a blender, process until smooth, and drink.

FRUITS AND VEGETABLES

1. Pineapple
2. Mango
3. Berries
4. Stone fruit (cherries, plums, or peaches)
5. Leafy greens
6. Avocado

LIQUIDS

1. Milk
2. Orange juice
3. Apple juice
4. Plant milk
5. Water
6. Coconut water

THICKENERS

1. Banana
2. Yogurt
3. Cottage cheese
4. Peanut butter
5. Chia seeds
6. Handful of nuts

EXTRAS

1. Dash of cinnamon
2. Honey
3. Black pepper
4. Pitted date
5. Grated ginger
6. Squeeze of lime juice

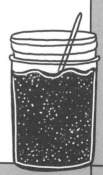

Hummus Among Us

Chickpeas are kind of magical. They're good whole, they're good smushed up, and the liquid they've been cooked and canned in—aquafaba—is a weirdly versatile egg white substitute. You can braise them like you would a tough cut of meat and have a satisfying vegetarian stew, you can frizzle them in hot olive oil to top a salad or soup, or you can just roast them in the oven and toss them in salt and pepper for a crunchy snack.

But if you have zero energy for any of that, chickpeas are still your friend. Not only are they a solid base for a bean salad, they are also the main ingredient in hummus, a dip substantial enough to fill you up and provide the base of a meal. Yes, a bowl of hummus counts as dinner.

HUMMUS FUNDAMENTALS

First, start with hummus. Do you have some in your fridge already? Cool, use that. Need to make some from scratch? No problem. There are many, many ways to make hummus. There's debate over whether canned or cooked-from-dry beans are better, whether to peel the chickpeas, what brand of tahini to use, and on and on. We're not going to deal with any of that, because the answer is that you should do whatever is easiest (hint: it's not peeling chickpeas!) and use whatever you have on hand. It's going to be good because it's going to be hummus.

You might already have a great hummus recipe, and if that's the case, by all means use it. If you don't, you can follow the one on page 114, or improvise and experiment with these basic principles!

When I make hummus, I add a clove or 2 of garlic and the juice of a lemon (or if no lemon is available, a tablespoon of white wine vinegar), and whip those together in a food processor. Then I dump in a whole can of chickpeas and as much tahini as I feel like using that day, usually about ¼ cup. If you like hummus and have the strength to source good tahini, it is, unfortunately, really worth it, but don't stress out too much if your tahini isn't fancy. If you don't have tahini, cashew butter, almond butter, or a couple teaspoons of sesame oil make a good substitute. Peanut butter works too, but it will make your hummus taste vaguely peanut butter-y—not necessarily a negative, but something worth noting. Then I throw in some olive oil and some spices, like a pinch of cumin or paprika, plus a pinch of salt, and blitz it. If you don't have chickpeas, use white beans—it won't technically be hummus, but it'll still be delicious.

You can make hummus just fine in a blender, too, or even a stand mixer if that's what you have (just make sure to use the paddle attachment, not the whisk, or it'll take forever). You can smash things together by hand, too, using a fork and some determination. It'll be more rustic and less creamy, but it'll taste good.

HOW TO EAT HUMMUS

So now you have hummus. What do you do with it? Easy. Slather it on some crackers or chips. Dunk in vegetables like carrots, celery, cucumbers, radishes, or raw broccoli. Spread it on toast. Plop some in a bowl and top with pickle slices, red onion, crumbled feta, and shredded rotisserie chicken and eat it for a meal. Cook some freezer meatballs and throw those on some hummus and add a handful of spinach. Mix it into cooked grains like rice, farro, or quinoa, and then throw a fried or soft-boiled egg on top. But you're probably going to shovel it into your mouth with a piece of pita bread, possibly while standing in the kitchen, and that's great too!

Do Exactly This: Hummus

Great hummus doesn't have to be fussy, and it doesn't have to arrive in a tub from the grocery store. It's also hearty enough that when eaten with pita, carrots, chips, or, honestly, just a spoon, it feels like either a robust snack or a light meal. Feel free to play around with herbs and spices in here too—a little spice blend or a hit of red pepper is really nice if you like things on the spicier side.

Ingredients

- About 2 tablespoons *lemon juice* (or 1 fresh lemon, squeezed)
- 1 clove *garlic*
- ¼ cup, or about 4 heaping spoonfuls, *tahini*
  - If you don't have tahini, *cashew butter* or *almond butter*
- 1 can *chickpeas*, drained
- ¼ cup olive oil, or about 4 big glugs
- 1 teaspoon *salt*
- 1 teaspoon *cumin*

Optional

- 1 teaspoon *paprika* or *smoked paprika*
- 1 to 2 tablespoons *ice water* (if needed to thin)

1. Find your food processor or blender, make sure the blade is settled in the bottom (so you don't have to futz with it after the hummus ingredients go into the bowl), and locate your ingredients. Put the lemon juice and garlic in the bottom of

the bowl first, and pulse the food processor until the garlic gets broken up a bit. (I learned this trick from Philadelphia's own king of hummus, Michael Solomonov, and it works to mellow out the raw garlic flavor—raw garlic packs way more punch than the cooked kind, so even if you spend your free time making memes about how you triple the garlic in every recipe, at least attempt this step with just a single clove. If it's not garlicky enough you can add more and tell me I'm wrong on the internet.)

2. Then add the tahini (or alternative) and pulse the food processor again until it combines. The mixture might look a little grainy right now, and that's OK. Add the chickpeas, olive oil, salt, cumin, and paprika (if using), and process them together until a smooth hummus-y looking dip forms. Use olive oil that you don't hate the taste of or it will return in the dip to haunt you.

3. When you're done processing, assess the texture. Is it too thick? Add 1 tablespoon ice water and pulse until it's incorporated. If it still seems too thick, add another tablespoon of ice water. Then taste the hummus. Add more salt or lemon juice if you'd like. Then scoop it into a container and eat it. It should last for a week in the fridge.

Grab-Bag Green Sauce

Here's a thing that happens to me all the time: I'm at the grocery store. The shelves of produce are dazzling—all bright colors and tender green leaves, hopes and ambitions of culinary delights to come. I grab a bunch of herbs and lettuces with grand ambitions for what I'll make that week. Then by the time I get back home, unpack, and put all the things I bought into their proper places, I'm too tired to deal with this fanciful meal and instead make something easy. I forget about the herbs until three days later when they are on the brink of becoming compost.

In this situation, I make what I think of as dirtbag pesto, or grab-bag green sauce. Depending on what I have around it can lean more toward a traditional basil pesto or more toward a salsa verde. Sometimes it comes out chimichurri-like, other times more like a green goddess dressing. But regardless, it tastes good and works great as a drizzle over a bowl of grains, a sauce for fried egg sandwiches, or a thing to dunk chicken nuggets into. It's also a good way to use herbs like cilantro, basil, parsley, and sage, as well as greens like spinach, arugula, and kale. And it's an incredibly simple formula.

THE FORMULA

Here's what you do. Put the sad wilted greens in the blender. (They don't *have* to be wilted, of course. If you have fresh herbs, those work too.) Then add our old faves acid and fat. You're gonna hunt for any acid that you have knocking around. Lemon juice, lime juice, apple cider vinegar, or white wine vinegar are my favorites for this particular application, but use whatever you've got. Put about a tablespoon of it in the blender with the greens. Then add about ¼ cup of something fatty like sour cream, Greek yogurt, mayonnaise, crème fraîche, labneh, or kefir. Add a good pinch of salt—that's roughly ¼ teaspoon. Then blend everything and taste it. Is it too sharp and acidic? Add more of your fatty dairy thing. Is it a little bland? Add a splash more of your acid and a little more salt. Is it too thick to pour? Add water, a tablespoon at a time, until it loosens up.

Want it to be more like a pesto thing, plus vegan to boot? Skip the dairy and use olive oil instead, and throw in a handful of nuts. Pine nuts are traditional in pesto but also wildly expensive, so unless I'm feeling wealthy, I usually end up using shelled pistachios or walnuts. If you are willing to make it not vegan, then throw in some grated parmesan or pecorino, blend and taste, and call it a day.

There's no limit to the green sauce. You can put in anchovies and olives for something briny and delicious. If you like things spicy, you can throw in a pinch of red pepper flakes or a dab of harissa or a spoonful of chili oil. A handful of feta is nice, and I always add at least a substantial sprinkle of ground black pepper in there. Green sauce can go spicy or mild, creamy or thin, chunky or smooth. It accommodates every preference, unless that preference is "no green things." If you have an immersion blender, you can make the sauce directly in a food storage container and throw it in the fridge. Use it as a spread, dip, or funky condiment. Thin it out with olive oil, and use it as a salad dressing. It'll last about a week.

Cottage Cheese Is Better Blended

Maybe you're already hip to the cottage cheese game, in which case you don't need me to tell you what a good thing it is to have some in the fridge for an easy meal or snack. It's got a ton of protein in it—I'm no nutritionist, but I know that when I go too long without eating protein I get extremely cranky—and you can dress it up in much the same way you can a bowl of oatmeal or yogurt. You can stir in some fruit and a little honey to sweeten it up, or chuck in a handful of chocolate chips and a swirl of peanut butter. You can take things in a savory direction and stir in salt, pepper, olive oil, and lemon juice. You can use it as a base for cut-up avocado, tomato, and cilantro. It's got a lot going for it, is what I'm saying.

The problem I've always had with cottage cheese isn't the flavor, which has the same nice dairy unctuousness as a piece of fresh mozzarella. It's the texture. I believe in dairy in all its forms, but there's something about the curds suspended in liquid that just doesn't do it for me. It's too lumpy. So until recently, I skipped cottage cheese in favor of Greek yogurt or oatmeal, which are smooth on purpose and lumpy on purpose, respectively. Until I learned a trick from, yes, Tik-Tok, that changed my entire cottage cheese game.

The trick is so easy it feels ridiculous: put it in the blender. Just dump that cottage cheese in your blender or food processor and blend it until it turns into one smooth texture. You don't need to add anything else—though sometimes I add salt and pepper, or a little hot sauce, lemon juice, and olive oil. All you do is pulse it together until it turns into more of a uniform pudding-looking thing than a lumpy curds thing. Then use it as the base of a bowl of whatever you want, or set it out with crackers and crudités as a makeshift easy dip.

The TikTok folks call this "whipped" cottage cheese, and you can also use that trick for other dairy products that you want to be more of a smooth dip and not chunks. Whipped cream cheese is excellent, and whipped feta is delicious—just throw feta in the blender with a drizzle of olive oil and process it until it turns into a dip. Beautiful.

Soup Part 2: Electric Soupaloo

I know, I know, we already talked about soup. There was a whole recipe and everything! What's the situation? The situation, my friends, is that blenders also make really easy, really hearty soup. If you like your soups a little on the thick but smooth side, blenders are where it's *at*. We're exiting the chicken noodle zone, and we're entering the butternut squash tier. Join me.

PUREED SOUP BASICS

A lot of thick soups—we're talking potato and leek, broccoli and cheddar, pumpkin, cauliflower, gazpacho, black bean—are really just purees, loosened a little bit with broth. That rules because blenders are excellent at making purees. The work you need to do is basically chopping, peeling (if necessary), and then cooking the vegetables. Sounds hard, but here's a secret: frozen vegetables are already chopped and peeled, and there's no reason why you shouldn't use them for soup. I usually roast them because all you do is cut up the vegetables (or, again, shake them out of the bag in your freezer), toss them in olive oil, and put them in a 400°F oven until they're cooked through (about 20 minutes, give or take, or 30 minutes if you're cooking from frozen).

Then put the vegetables in the blender. Add broth, about a cup, or if you don't have broth, water and a splash of wine. If you don't have wine, just water is honestly fine. Blend it until the whole thing turns into a smooth paste. Add more liquid, ¼ cup at a time, until it gets to the consistency of soup you like. Taste it. Add salt and pepper, or more spices if you're feeling creative. Cumin and coriander are good go-tos for vegetable puree soups, and so are those spice blends I'm always going on about. A little bit of acid is nice—a splash of wine or a squeeze of lemon. Then you'll probably want to heat it up. If it's for just you, you can put it in a bowl and microwave it 30 seconds at a time, stirring between intervals, until it's hot enough. If it's for a group, dumping it in a stockpot and heating it on the stove is probably your best bet. Follow our previous protocol about topping it with crunchy things or cheese and boom, soup.

If roasting a vegetable sounds like an ordeal, I hear you. Here's a soup that only requires opening of cans.

Do Exactly This: Black Bean Blender Soup

Black beans from a can are already a simple, if somewhat bleak, meal. Throwing them in a blender with a few more ingredients, like a jar of salsa, gives the whole affair a little extra flavor and a few extra vegetables, and who could be mad at that?

Ingredients
- 2 15-ounce cans **black beans**
- 1 jar **salsa**
- 1½ to 2 cups chicken or vegetable **broth** (or throw in one can or half a carton, probably, depending on how it's packaged, or use bouillon)
- 1 teaspoon **cumin**
- ½ teaspoon **coriander**
- **Salt and pepper**

Optional
- Pinch of **red pepper flakes**

1. Find your blender or food processor, and line up your ingredients. You're also going to need a pot to warm the soup, so find that. Drain the can of black beans, then dump them into the blender along with the salsa, about 1½ cups broth, the spices, and a good pinch of salt. Blend until the ingredients come together in a uniform texture, usually after about 1 minute. Assess the texture of the soup. Does it look like soup or black bean spread? If it's more of a spread, add ¼ cup more broth and blend again. Keep doing that, ¼ cup at a time, until it reaches the right consistency. If it feels like soup to you—good news, it's soup.

2. Taste it. Add more salt, pepper, or red pepper flakes (if you're using them) to your liking. Then pour the soup into the pot and heat, stirring occasionally, until the soup starts bubbling gently. Cut off the heat, ladle the soup into bowls, and eat. A dollop of sour cream or a sprig of cilantro goes great with this soup if you like that and have it on hand. If you don't, skip it.

Simple Sauces

Easy sauces are the living room rugs of mealtime—they tie everything together. You can have the most random assemblage of vegetables, protein, and starch, and with a good sauce, suddenly it's a cohesive meal. You can, of course, just use something from your condiment collection, but you can also throw together one of my following list of simple sauces for way more sense of accomplishment with only a little more effort.

THREE-INGREDIENT SAUCE FORMULAS

You can make any of these in the blender, or just whisk them together with a fork. If the sauce is too thick, loosen it up with a teaspoon of water at a time until it reaches the consistency you're looking for. You can make more than the formula calls for—just keep the ratios the same.

Stir-fry sauce: 4 tablespoons soy sauce + 1 tablespoon sriracha + 1 tablespoon brown sugar

Sauce for sheet pan vegetables: 2 tablespoons tahini (or 1 tablespoon peanut butter and 1 tablespoon water) + 2 tablespoons hoisin sauce + 2 tablespoons water

Dip for vegetables: ¼ cup mayonnaise + 2 tablespoons chili crisp + 2 teaspoons apple cider vinegar

Miso dressing: 1 tablespoon miso + 1 tablespoon olive oil + 1 tablespoon apple cider vinegar

Umami sauce for grain bowls: 1 tablespoon miso + 2 tablespoons tahini + 2 tablespoons lemon juice

Green goddess-y dressing: 2 tablespoons yogurt + 2 tablespoons pesto + 1 tablespoon olive oil

Sort-of cocktail sauce: ¼ cup ketchup + 1 tablespoon horseradish + ½ tablespoon Worcestershire sauce

Blue cheese sauce: equal parts blue cheese + Greek yogurt or mayo

Thai-inspired sauce: 1 tablespoon brown sugar + 1 tablespoon fish sauce + 1 tablespoon lime juice

Easy dessert sauce: equal parts jam + whipped cream

BUFFALO IT

Maybe the undisputed king of simple sauces is buffalo sauce. All you need for buffalo sauce is hot sauce and butter. Yes, actually. That's it. You heat equal amounts of butter and your favorite hot sauce—I love Frank's Red Hot for this, but I have used Tabasco, Crystal, and some random challenge hot sauce that promises to ruin your day. I start with ¼ cup of each, which is 4 tablespoons if you are going by the butter wrapper ruler. Melt the butter and add the hot sauce, and swirl it together until it combines. Then taste it.

Is it too hot for your liking? Add more butter. Not hot enough? Add more hot sauce. Now use it to coat anything you want. Wings, of course, but also chunks of tofu, roasted cauliflower or broccoli, shrimp, or cooked frozen chicken tenders. It makes a killer dip when swirled into yogurt or sour cream. It's also a great dunk for tater tots or french fries, and equally great drizzled over leftover pizza. You can toss popcorn in it and feel happy with your life choices. You can swirl it into eggs for a spicy treat, or spoon it over ice cream if you're freaky like that. You can buffalo anything you want if you put your mind to it. And also? Maybe you *should*.

Cook Something

How to eat when you have the wherewithal to fry, slice, chop, or mash—but not too much

Do you have the energy and time to chop, slice, mash, or roast, as long as all of those activities are optimized for someone who is so, so sleepy? First of all, congratulations, that's no mean feat. Second, welcome, this is the chapter for you. Here are the things that require a knife and a skillet or oven, but are still, I promise, really, really easy. They are the kind of recipes that give you the afterglow of victory for not ordering takeout, but leave a minimum of dishes in your wake, come together with minimal effort, and may not require you to go to the grocery store even once (in fact, you'll find some handy tips in here for using the leftovers you already have around). We've got noodles, we've got dumplings, we've got fried rice and stir-fry, we've got the kind of casserole that you can throw together with whatever weird things you have knocking around in your freezer and eat for a week.

Eggs Part Two: The Eggening

Slapping an egg on something is a great way to add protein and a general sense of pomp and ceremony to something that would otherwise just be "leftovers" or "a piece of bread." If you don't eat eggs, great news—you can skip this section, because there are easy vegan egg substitutes that come in a carton and you can just follow the directions. But if you're using the kind that come out of a chicken, read on to level up your game.

FRIED EGGS, NO SNOT

As discussed (see page 99), I believe very strongly in cooking eggs in the microwave when you simply cannot deal with a pan and its ramifications. But if you *can* deal with a pan, it does have certain advantages. Namely, it's the best way to get an egg that has that coveted crispy edge that's so nice on toast, particularly when coupled with the liquid of a good yolk. Eggs are self-saucing and I think that's beautiful!

You probably already have a good idea of how to cook a fried egg (it is, at heart, not complicated—put an egg in a pan with oil or butter and add heat). But maybe, like me, you run into the problem that the bottom is crispy but the egg white on top hasn't quite set, and you don't want the bottom to burn, but also there's basically nothing worse than biting into the snot-like tendrils of a not-cooked egg white. I'm sorry, I said what I said. Here's the solution for cooking an egg that is always crisped through: steam.

I learned this trick from Julia Turshen's lovely cookbook *Small Victories*, one I leaf through all the time for inspiration, and I've never gone back. Start with a pan that has a lid—nonstick is easy mode, but seasoned cast-iron or stainless steel works too—and set it on medium-high heat. Drizzle in some olive oil (about a tablespoon) or chuck in a knob of butter (again, about a tablespoon but I'm not the butter police, you can use more). Then crack an egg into the pan. If you're worried about breaking the yolk, crack the egg into another container, like a small bowl or glass, and gently pour it into the pan.

Let the egg sizzle in the pan until the edges are looking browned and crispy. Then get a little bit of water—a tablespoon or 2 if you want to be precise, but I usually just put a little in my cupped hand— pour it in the pan, and put the lid on. It'll hiss and steam effusively, and that is exactly what you want. The steam collected under the top of the lid will gently cook the top of the egg so you don't have any mucus-y egg white, but it won't harden the tender inner yolk. After a minute, remove the lid. You should have an egg that has a crispy bottom, a set but custardy yolk, and no weird uncooked white. Slide it out of the pan onto a plate—or a pile of greens, a bowl of grains, a slice of pizza, whatever—and eat it. Done.

OMELET WITH ANYTHING

Eggs are extremely good at turning a haphazard bunch of ingredients into a meal. Quiches, frittatas, omelets—they're all just ways of encasing things in egg so you can eat them more easily. It's like a salad, and eggs are the gelatinous dressing pulling it all together.

You can really add most anything to an omelet—chopped-up pizza, blue cheese, crumbled chips, a handful of torn-up cold cuts, some roasted vegetables that have been sadly lingering in the fridge—but there are a few caveats that will help you on the way.

Preparing to omelet

First, the ingredients should be pretty dry. A lot of extra liquid will thin out your eggs in a way that can be unpleasant and lead to unintentional egg drop soup. Second, your ingredients won't be in the pan long enough to really cook anything through, so no raw vegetables that take longer than a couple minutes to cook. Raw potatoes? No. Don't do it. Crunchy in a bad way. Use leftover fries, tots, or any cooked potatoes if you want potato in there. But frozen peas? Arugula? Well-drained diced tomatoes? Sure, yes, fine, love it. Third, limit your omelet fillings to ½ cup. That doesn't sound like a lot, I know, but if you add too much, you're essentially going to have a Dagwood sandwich–style omelet. Which doesn't sound bad! It's just a different vibe. Fourth, if you want the fillings in the omelet to be hot, heat them up in the microwave before adding to the eggs. They won't be in the pan long enough to totally reheat. So if you're, say, adding cut-up french fries, make sure they're at least at room temperature before you add them to the omelet. Otherwise, you're going to have a cold french fry omelet. Fine! Not a disaster! Just not ideal.

Also if you're keeping tabs on the technical aspects, we're going to go with an American diner-style omelet here, meaning that you can brown it, stuff it with a bunch of weird things, and not worry about the texture being set *just so*. A French omelet is its own thing and we salute it, just from far away, on our own shores.

Omelets away!

So here's what you're going to do. Get your fillings out, and if they're not already, cut them into roughly bite-size chunks. If you're using, say, leftover buffalo wings or chicken fingers, cut those up. If you're using cherry tomatoes, halve them, and if you're using a handful of arugula or spinach, that's fine, it can chill. If you want a cheese in there, make sure it's one that's shredded up so it'll melt quickly, or one you don't mind being less than totally melted, like crumbled feta or blue cheese. American cheese rules here. I'm not going to stop extolling the virtues of American cheese.

Then crack 3 eggs into a bowl. Add a pinch of salt and mix the eggs together with a fork until they become a single egg blob, with no yolk or whites separated. Don't worry about it being whipped perfectly, just get them into a relatively homogeneous mixture.

Heat a frying pan (nonstick is easiest, if you have one) over medium-high heat for about a minute, and then add a tablespoon of olive oil or butter. Swirl the oil or butter around the pan so it coats the bottom. Again, it doesn't have to be perfect, just sort of even distribution is what we're going for. Then dump your eggs into the pan, and use a spatula to nudge them around the pan so that it looks like they're in an even layer. You can also pick up the pan and swirl the eggs around it to get an even layer, which I personally find very satisfying, but if it's intimidating to you, stick with the spatula. Then leave the egg to cook for a minute or 2 until it's set at the bottom but still looking wet at the top.

Sprinkle or spoon your fillings over the top of the egg, trying your best to get them even, but not stressing too much if it doesn't work out quite that way. It's all getting mushed up in your stomach anyway. Then clap a lid on the pan for a minute—just like the fried eggs, the steam from the liquid will help cook the top of the eggs gently, and it'll soften up those fillings and melt cheese if you have cheese in the mix. Take the lid off, and fold the omelet in half by wedging a spatula under one side and flipping it over the other side. (Again, just not a big deal if you don't fold it exactly in half—it will still be good.) Then slip it onto a plate. Done. Amazing. Easy. Food.

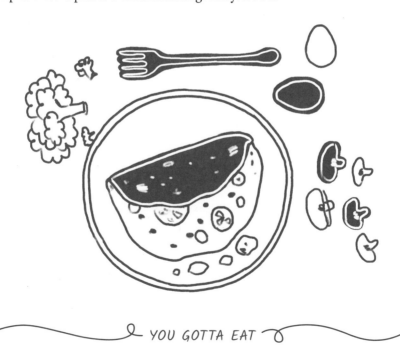

YOU OUGHTA FRITTATA

Omelets are great for one or two people, but if you have a crowd to feed, standing over the stove and making individual eggs for people is a pain. (That is, unless you love doing short-order cook at the Hilton brunch cosplay. And if you do, god bless but you are probably not reading this book.) A frittata is basically all the great things about an omelet—you can clean out the fridge and throw in a bunch of left-overs or about-to-die vegetables without worrying too much whether they "go," because the eggs bring everything together. The difference is that it uses the oven instead of the stove, and it's a larger dish that you can slice and serve. It also is wildly inexpensive to make, and takes about twenty minutes from the moment you think "Hey, I'll make a frittata" to an actual frittata being on the table.

Frittata theory

A frittata is not a quiche, which is a similar idea but requires a pie crust—a whole other finicky world that you simply do not have to deal with. A quiche is kind of like a pie but the pie is egg, plus dairy, plus whatever things you have knocking around that sound good with eggs, and a frittata is also that but minus the crust. Also, it's a fun word to say.

Some but not all of the principles of an omelet apply here. Fillings need to be cut into bite-size chunks, and they should still be dry and not liquidy. But unlike an omelet, you don't need to heat the fillings beforehand. I still wouldn't throw in a raw potato or onion—those aren't gonna cook and they'll be crunchy in a bad way—but you don't need to worry about reheating chicken fingers or cut-up Bagel Bites or whatever else you're using. The other thing is that cheese is pretty standard in a frittata, rather than optional like in an omelet. But here you can use cheese that's a little more stubborn to melt—like brie or gruyère. Just make sure you grate it or cut it up into bite-size chunks.

Also, because a frittata uses more eggs and sets around the fillings, rather than the eggs setting first before fillings are added as in an omelet, you can use way more stuff in one. Like *way* more. We're talking 2 to 3 cups of filling. Bacon, cheese, spinach, broccoli, ham, meatballs, cherry tomatoes, leftover tandoori chicken, yes, yes, yes. Frittatas may sound fancy, but they can accommodate all your fridge scrap dreams.

Frittatas in practice

So here's what you do. Locate an oven-safe pan (most pans are oven-safe, but many nonstick pans can't go into the oven, so if you're worried, avoid nonstick). I usually use my 10-inch cast-iron skillet for this, but if you have something smaller or larger, that's cool, you'll just want to adjust the number of eggs you use. If you're using a 10-inch skillet, you'll want 6 eggs, ¼ cup of milk, cream, half-and-half, or nondairy milk, and 2 cups of filling, cut into bite-size pieces. You'll also want 1 cup of cheese, shredded, grated, or chunked into roughly even crumbles. For a 12-inch skillet, add 2 more eggs and 2 tablespoons extra milk.

Preheat the oven to 400°F, and locate your ingredients. Crack all the eggs into a bowl, add the milk (or substitute), 2 pinches of salt, and a couple good cracks or shakes of black pepper in there. Whisk the eggs together so that there are no distinguishable yolks and white parts. Then get your oven-safe skillet out. Put it on the stove over medium heat, and put in a tablespoon or 2 of olive oil. After about a minute, when the oil is hot, add your fillings (not including your cheese) to the skillet. Then add the cheese to the top of the fillings and pour the egg mixture over that. It's fine if the eggs don't totally cover the fillings. It'll look like a big soupy mess, and that is just fine.

Turn the heat on the stove off, and transfer the pan with the egg mess to the oven.

The trick with a frittata is to not overcook it, because then things get rubbery and the eggs can start to break down and extrude liquid. If that happens it's not the end of the world, but if you want to avoid it, just pull the frittata out of the oven when it still looks a little jiggly and wet—kind of like getting that extra-gooey center in a pan of brownies. Eggs will keep cooking a bit after you pull them from the oven, too. In my oven, baking a frittata for 14 minutes is just about perfect, but in general I'd aim for 12 to 15 minutes. If you're feeling unsure about your oven and frittata prowess, bake it for 10 minutes and then check on it—if the center looks set, even if it's still a little wet, it's done. If the center looks liquidy, give it another 2 minutes.

Take the frittata out and let it cool down for 5 minutes before you slice it and serve it. If you're feeling spicy, you can flip it out onto a plate, but you can serve as is from the skillet if you'd rather not risk it. If you have some herbs, you can sprinkle those on top. Potato chip crumbs are a great finisher for omelets and frittatas too (if you don't believe me watch the second season of *The Bear*), but you don't need to do any of that. A little green salad on the side is a classic frittata accompaniment and can make it feel more like a meal, but a slice of cold frittata, straight from the fridge, eaten over the sink, is equally as classic.

EGG IN THE MIDDLE

You can just make fried eggs and eat them with toast, and that is delicious and great. Or you can make things a little whimsical and fry an egg *inside* a piece of toast. This dish has a bunch of different names—toad in a hole, egg in a basket, egg in a hole—but basically all it consists of is a piece of buttered bread with a hole cut in it, and an egg plonked in that hole and cooked. (In England, toad in a hole has other components like sausages and Yorkshire pudding batter, but whatever, we won the Revolutionary War.) The reason to cook an egg like this is mostly whimsy—it looks cool and feels like a satisfying little treat. If it feels too fussy, skip it and make eggs another easier way (like in the microwave—see pages 99–100).

But if you're up for a little bit of whimsy, then making an egg in a hole couldn't be simpler. Basically you just need a slice of bread, some butter, and an egg. First, butter your bread on both sides. If you don't have butter around, use mayonnaise—it works, trust me. Then, take a cookie cutter or drinking glass and cut a round hole in the middle of the bread. Don't throw away the little bread round you just made— you're going to fry that too, and use it for dipping.

Grab a skillet that has a lid and heat it over medium heat. (If it's not a nonstick skillet, add a bit of oil or butter to coat the pan, too.) Plonk in both pieces of bread, the one with a hole in it and the round hole part, and fry them on both sides until they're golden brown and everything smells buttery and irresistible. Remove the round piece of toast from the pan. Then gently crack an egg into the hole you made in the bread. If you're nervous about getting eggshell in there or accidentally scrambling the yolk, crack the egg into a bowl or measuring cup first, and then pour the egg into the bread hole. Sprinkle some salt and pepper over the egg and toast. Put a lid over the pan and let the egg sizzle and cook for 2 minutes. If you like the yolk to be cooked through, rather than runny, add another minute. Remove the lid and check out the egg in the hole. Does it look cooked through? Great! You're done. Not yet? Sprinkle a tiny amount of water—run your hand under the tap and use what clings to your fingertips—into the pan, and clap the lid back on for another minute.

Aw, Sheet (Pan Meals)

God, I love sheet pans. Yes, they are simply large slabs of aluminum with a rim, but they're also some of the most useful, least expensive pieces of cooking equipment I own. You can pile a bunch of tools and ingredients on one to bring them outside to the grill. You can serve things directly off them and claim that it is because your aesthetic is rustic, not because you couldn't possibly be bothered to transfer food to another plate that you just have to wash later. And they're also a way to make a largely hands-off, anything-goes kind of meal. You can throw a bunch of ingredients on a sheet pan, put it in the oven, and then watch an episode of television for thirty minutes, or deal with the teetering pile of laundry, or calm down a raucous toddler, or whatever else while it cooks—no hovering over the stove. It's also usually easy to clean up after—typically I just need to wash a bowl, a knife, a cutting board, and the sheet pan itself. Incredible.

You can cook basically anything on a sheet pan in the oven, barring things that are largely liquid, or things that need to be cooked in liquid. (Do not attempt sheet pan soup, or sheet pan spaghetti.) But a sheet pan isn't necessarily the *best* tool for every kind of meal. Where it really excels, though, is a particular kind of super-easy mélange meal that requires very little thought, uses up what you've got in the house, and feeds a family (or one person for several days).

It's also a great way to transfer energy from your current self to your future self. If you have a little extra time and willpower, you can roast up a bunch of vegetables on a sheet pan, put them in the fridge, and then use them for sandwiches (pages 21 and 61) or soups (pages 29 and 119) or put them in a bowl with green sauce (page 115) and an easy egg (page 99) for a later low-effort meal.

When it comes to making sheet pan meals that are easy and delicious, I operate on a couple of cooking principles and go culinary off-roading. Here are a few simple steps that you need to keep in mind for sheet pan success.

FIND A PROTEIN

I like to use salmon, chicken thighs, cubed tofu, or chickpeas. Sausages and meatballs, whether pork, poultry, or beef, also work well here. I wouldn't do pork or beef that hadn't been processed into meatballs or sausage, because roasting isn't the ideal cooking situation for those. Tempeh or seitan would also work. I also love adding slabs of feta to a sheet pan meal—it gets browned on the outside but creamy on the inside. If you have a large cut of meat, it's easier to cut it into pieces so it cooks more quickly. Chunks or slices of chicken breast, for example, cook a lot quicker than a whole cut of chicken. That's important because otherwise you'll end up with vegetables that are overdone by the time the meat cooks through. On the other hand, whole salmon filets or chicken thighs, because they're usually compact, work well here. If you don't have anything on hand, you can skip the protein part and just dress up your roasted vegetables later with some goat cheese or a fried egg (page 127).

FIND SOME VEGETABLES

Avoid things that are really watery, like salad greens or cucumber—if you have those on hand, you can still use them, but they go on at the same time as garnishes. Look for heartier guys that benefit from roasting, like brussels sprouts, sweet potatoes, zucchini, onions, broccoli, broccolini, cauliflower, eggplant, bok choy, squash, green beans, peppers, asparagus, or potatoes. I also really like using cherry tomatoes, or whole tomatoes cut up, for a little pop of acidic brightness. Cut up the vegetables until they're in roughly even bite-size pieces, which will help them cook more evenly, and also save you from having to do some cutting up later. (Many grocery stores sell roasting vegetables already cut!) If it's something that's already a bite-size piece, like cherry tomatoes or brussels sprouts, just cut it in half. For onions, I slice them rather than mince them, and for long guys like green beans and asparagus, I usually just break them in half. Bear in mind that denser vegetables, like potatoes and turnips, need to cook longer than tomatoes or broccoli—you can fix that by cutting them up smaller (the smaller you cut them, the faster they'll cook through).

USE SOME OIL

Once you have your chunks of vegetables and protein going, toss them in a bowl and add some olive oil, salt, and pepper. You want enough olive oil so that it coats the vegetables, but not so much that there's a big puddle of oil at the bottom of the bowl. Add a couple glugs and toss the vegetables and protein, and if they don't seem coated, repeat. You can also use canola or avocado oil for this, whatever you have on hand.

GET SPICY

While you're tossing the bits of vegetables and protein in the oil, add some spices so they can get tossed around too. I like to add cumin and a pinch of red pepper flakes, and maybe some smoked paprika. But you can experiment with whatever you have. Taco seasoning, curry powder, cajun seasoning, chili powder, that thing your uncle gave you for Christmas that he promises is a secret proprietary spice blend that's great on barbecue, whatever other spice mix you have knocking around—go for it! Anything that you think would taste good can go here. Add a teaspoon or 2 at a time and toss the vegetables around in the oil and spice mix so that there's a little bit on all of the pieces. Herbs work here too, but go for the woodier ones, like rosemary, thyme, or oregano, if you have them.

DON'T OVERCROWD

Once you've tossed the bits and pieces of your meal in oil and spices, dump them out on a sheet pan. Some people use parchment paper or foil to line their sheet pans for easy cleaning, and I respect that, but I skip it, because I find that a bare sheet pan makes things crispier. Look at how crowded the pan is. You want everything to be in one layer—it's fine for the vegetables to touch each other, but avoid a lot of overlapping. Does it feel like it's overflowing? Just split the meal onto two sheet pans. You can also cook the vegetables on one sheet pan and the protein on another, or separate different kinds of vegetables onto two sheet pans, like brussels sprouts on one and sweet potato chunks on another. (This is also a handy approach if you've got one element you're worried about cooking too fast or too slow, like a piece of fish.) The more crowded your sheet pan is, the more the vegetables are going to steam rather than roast, which means less of a browned exterior. That's completely fine and edible either way, it just depends on what you prefer.

COOK

I usually set my oven at 400°F and check on the pan for 20 minutes, and then at 5-minute intervals after that. I pull the pan out when the contents look done to me, or when the vegetables yield to a fork without too much resistance and the protein is a little browned at the edges and doesn't look raw in the middle when I cut into it to check.

FINISHING TOUCHES

Once your sheet pan materials are cooked through, you can eat them as is, or add a little extra touch. I like squeezing a lemon or drizzling a little bit of red wine vinegar over everything to bring out the flavors.

If you have tender herbs like cilantro, basil, or mint, you can sprinkle them on after the contents are out of the oven. You can also mix in smooshed-up green olives (no pits, though) for some pops of briny flavor, or sprinkle some arugula or cut-up cucumber on there for a nice little bit of freshness and flavor. Eat the sheet pan meal as is, or ladle it over cooked grains. You can also dress it with one of our simple not-secret sauces (page 121), or not bother and just eat it as is. You can eat it directly off the sheet if you want. No one can stop you.

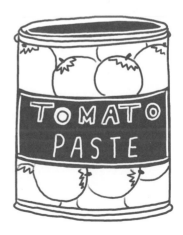

Kitchen Shears, for When Knives Are Too Hard

There are times when the act of fetching a cutting board and knife seems impossibly hard. For me it's one of those tasks that amasses a great deal of friction even when I'm feeling otherwise fine about cooking, like getting a plate for my silly little snack when a square of paper towel works fine and eliminates having to wash the dish later. When that happens, I turn to my kitchen shears.

Cutting up herbs with a knife? No thank you. I just take out my kitchen shears and snip the herbs into smaller pieces. (This works particularly well for soft herbs whose tender stems are OK to eat, such as parsley, cilantro, or basil.) Taking a knife to a billion cherry tomatoes? Nah, I'll just use the shears to snip them in half. Cutting up whole tomatoes from a tin can be horrible, and draining them and chopping on a cutting board or even smashing them in a bowl creates more mess that you eventually have to clean up. Instead, I just open the can and use shears in the can to roughly cut the tomatoes up. You can cut up bone-less chicken for a stir-fry, chunk beef for a stew, or slice Italian sausage for a pasta dish.

I've found that shears are also wonderful if you aren't

confident in your knife skills, or if you're in a situation in which using a chef's knife is dangerous, onerous, or unpleasant. Kids can usually handle shears a little more easily than a chef's knife, and when I'm in someone else's kitchen and the knives are either occupied, in bizarre novelty shapes, or dull, shears come in handy to do a lot of the cutting-related kitchen tasks. You probably already have some shears, but if you don't, my very favorite kitchen scissors are trauma shears, the kind they use at hospitals to cut clothes off patients. They're strong, sharp, dishwashable, and inexpensive, and many of them have a carabiner in the handle, which is just cool. I got hip to this off-label use of trauma shears thanks to my friend Liz, a plastic surgeon, who uses them in their kitchen and in the trauma bay—but not the same pair, obviously. I bought mine from Amazon in a set of three, and I've never looked back.

Send Noodles

If this is not your first Struggle Cooking rodeo, you already know how to survive on packets of ramen and boxes of mac and cheese. If you've read this book so far, you even know how to make those prepackaged meals a little celebratory and fun. (If you missed that part, see page 44 for ramen and page 49 for mac.) But did you know that for *barely* any more energy expenditure, you can cook a pasta dish that will taste even better *and* make you feel accomplished?

FROZEN RAVIOLI, MVP

I grew up on store-bought refrigerated ravioli as a staple easy meal, for when my busy parents had to feed three children with a minimum of fuss and dissent. As an adult, I've often leaned on refrigerated or frozen tortellini or ravioli with some modicum of protein already included for an easy meal. You can get a whole spectrum of fillings in these little stuffed pastas, from veal to lobster to pumpkin to roasted mushroom.

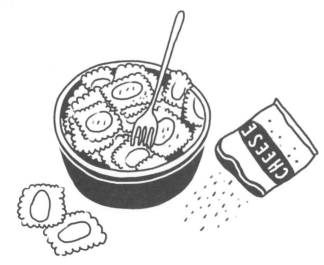

The classic way of cooking premade ravioli—and the way I grew up with—is to dump it in boiling water, wait the assigned number of minutes on the package, strain it, and eat it with a drizzle of olive oil and a showering of parmesan, or with a pat of butter and some black pepper in there. It's a great method, and it gets something on the table quickly, without much fuss.

But thanks to Deb Perelman—the brilliant mind behind Smitten Kitchen and someone whose recipes are constantly on my "I should make this" list on my phone—a few years ago I realized that you can treat frozen or refrigerated stuffed pasta like they're tiny potstickers, which means you don't even need boiling water to cook them through. It also means you can get satisfying crispy edges on the pasta shapes, something that offers a nice textural contrast in what is otherwise a bowl of mushy food. The following flexible recipe-ish thing is a riff on Perelman's excellent crispy tortellini with peas and prosciutto, a recipe I've adapted to my own purposes with whatever I have around. It's often a lifesaver when I'm too hungry to think but remember that I have frozen ravioli (or tortellini) on hand—it's a perfect meal for two, or a meal for one plus a portion of leftovers for lunch the next day.

CRISP IT UP

Here's what you do: Take out a pan that has a lid, and locate your pasta and a small vessel for water. Heat the pan over medium-high, and drizzle in some olive oil. Aim for a tablespoon or so—it doesn't have to be exact, just enough to coat the bottom of the pan without any trouble. After a minute or so, when the oil is hot, dump in your frozen or refrigerated pasta and arrange them into a single layer on the pan. Let them hang out for a couple minutes—like 2 or 3 actual minutes—getting browned and crispy on the bottom, and then stir them around to make sure that they're cooking evenly. Don't worry if not every single piece of pasta gets browned, you're just looking for enough of them to be crispy-edged to be tasty.

At this point, if you want, you can throw in a handful of frozen vegetables for extra heft, like our old pal frozen peas, or some frozen spinach, broccoli, or cauliflower. If you have some baby spinach hanging out in the fridge, a handful of that will do great here too. If you don't have those things or you don't want to, skip that part.

Then get about ¼ cup of water and a lid for the pan. You can eyeball it if you want—it doesn't have to be precise. Pour the water into the pan, clap on the lid, and turn the heat slightly down to medium. If you're like, wait, Margaret, this is the same trick as the egg thing (page 127)—yes! Correct. It's a good trick for anything you want to be crispy but also cooked all the way through. There will be a lot of hissing and a great plume of steam trapped under the lid. That's exactly what you want to happen; do not panic. The steam will finish cooking the pasta (and cook the frozen vegetables through if you're using them). Leave the pan to do its steam thing for about 5 minutes. If the steam appears to have all evaporated before then, add a little bit more water. Then take the lid off the pan so any excess water can sizzle off, and turn the heat off.

DRESS IT UP

This is a great situation as is, but you probably also want some kind of easy sauce here, or at least I always do. A drizzle of red wine vinegar or a squeeze of lemon juice does a good job of giving contrast to the starchiness of the pasta. Plunk in a few tablespoons of sour cream, ricotta, cream cheese, mascarpone, or crème fraîche and stir for an easy creamy sauce. If you have pesto hanging out in your fridge, drizzle a little extra olive oil in the pan and add a few tablespoons of the pesto, stirring it around the warm pan so it loosens up and coats the pasta. You can also add 2 tablespoons of butter and 2 tablespoons of tomato paste, again stirring to coat everything and mix them together, for our easy riff on tomato sauce. Or, if you want a cacio e pepe vibe, drop in a tablespoon of butter, a handful of parmesan, and a bunch of black pepper, again making sure it's evenly distributed. The seasonings within the ravioli vary, but I almost always need to add a little extra salt and pepper on the top.

Crispy bits of pork, such as bacon, prosciutto, or cubed Spam, also work really well in this dish. You'll just want to cook them before you make the pasta and add them back into the dish once the pasta is done steaming. You can use the same skillet to cook the meat in, and then use the drippings from the fat to crisp up the pasta rather than using olive oil. That's recycling.

Premade Gnocchi Is No Jokey

If you hear the word *gnocchi* and recoil, listen, I get it. I once went over to a friend's house at 8:30 for dinner. Except when I arrived, I realized that I was supposed to help make the dinner, and the dinner was gnocchi from scratch, *and* the dubious internet recipe that we were working with indicated that it would only take like, thirty seconds to make. Needless to say: absolutely not. Handmade pasta is not a project to launch into when you're feeling faint and irritable from hunger, let alone handmade pasta that first requires you to cook potatoes for a dough. We ate dinner at, like, midnight, after much troubleshooting and general grumpiness and rejected offers to order pizza. It was fine, and yes, we are still friends, but it was not an experience I'd overall recommend.

You know what will never betray you like that? Store-bought gnocchi. Maybe that's a section of pasta land that you've never ventured into, but let me urge you to stop at that point in the pasta aisle (or the freezer aisle) once more. Some premade gnocchi is sold frozen, but you can also buy packets of them that are shelf-stable that can hang out for a very long time in your pantry, awaiting their day in the sun.

THE JOY OF GNOCCHI

The person who really opened my eyes to the joy of gnocchi is Ali Slagle, whose cookbook *I Dream of Dinner (So You Don't Have To)* is one that is extremely sauce-spattered and dog-eared in my kitchen, my highest compliment. Slagle loves premade gnocchi, but not just as something you can boil and sauce, although of course you can. The gnocchi-redefining idea Slagle introduced me to is that (like ravioli) gnocchi can be crisped up. This gives you another nice textural element to your dish, and it avoids the problem that I often have with gnocchi, which is that it's mostly a bowl of flavorful mushes. No shade to mush, but I just want something in there to be a little al dente, you know?

When you crisp gnocchi up, either in a pan or in the oven, they become less pasta and more perfect little roasted potato pockets, chewy with a golden crust on the exterior. Throw those into a sauce and you'll be an even happier camper. And, hey, what's that, you can make them on a sheet pan, too? Wow, life is grand.

GNOCCHI VARIATIONS

You can throw gnocchi in with your other sheet pan standards, and experiment with it as you like. There aren't a ton of rules here. What if you hate sheet pans, or you use your oven to store sweaters, or it's already too hot in your house? No problem. You can crisp up gnocchi in a frying pan, too. Just warm a swirl of olive oil in a medium-hot skillet for a minute, then put the gnocchi on it in a single layer. Try not to move them around too much for the first 3 to 5 minutes, which will encourage them to toast on the bottom. When they're brown on the bottom, they're done.

Then just add an easy sauce, and a vegetable if you feel up to it. Frozen peas, yes, for sure. A handful of baby spinach, or some arugula. The easiest sauce is just melting some butter in the pan with the gnocchi and adding in some capers until they sizzle and brown. But you can try all kinds of easy sauces, like the ones we touched on earlier (page 122). Buffalo gnocchi? Who is gonna be mad about that?

I like the following recipe because it has the convenient aspect of saucing itself, thanks to the tomatoes that will roast and then burst, and the shallots, which add a nice allium zing to the operation. Spice as you see fit—I've used cumin and smoked paprika with success. You can leave the feta out and just add a shower of parmesan or pecorino at the end. You can also throw some smashed whole cloves of garlic in the mix to roast, if you're a big garlic fan, like my husband is. Finish with a handful of greens if you have them, and that's kind of all you need. It also doesn't leave that many dishes to wash—a knife, a cutting board, a mixing bowl, a sheet pan, and a measuring spoon and cup if you want to be precise, plus the bowls and forks you eat it with.

Do Exactly This: Crispy Gnocchi and Tomatoes
This recipe harnesses two of my favorite things: throwing everything on a sheet pan rather than cooking individual components,

and crispy pasta. As good as regular pasta is, crispy pasta is even better. To quote "Uptown Funk": "Don't believe me? Just watch."

Ingredients

- 2 pints (about 4 cups) cherry tomatoes
- 1 pound dried or frozen gnocchi
- ¼ cup olive oil, plus more to taste
- Salt and pepper
- 1 6-ounce block feta, cut into roughly 1-inch slices

Optional

- 1 shallot or ½ red onion
- ¼ to ½ teaspoon red pepper flakes
- Handful of spinach or arugula

1. Find a sheet pan, a cutting board, a big mixing bowl, a knife, and your ingredients, and turn your oven on to 400°F. Slice or snip up your shallot, if using. If you don't have a shallot, a red onion will work too, and if you don't have either or just don't like onions, skip it. Don't worry about getting the pieces super thin—just make them as regularly sized as you can. Toss the shallots, tomatoes, and gnocchi in a mixing bowl with the olive oil, 2 pinches of salt, and about 10 grinds or shakes of black pepper. Add the red pepper flakes too, if you'd like.

2. Toss them around until everything looks evenly coated with oil, salt, and pepper, and dump them out onto a sheet pan. Try to make sure that everything is evenly spread out—if the

ingredients are on top of each other too much, the gnocchi won't crisp, which would be perfectly edible but, you know, not crispy. If there's too much on the sheet pan for that to happen, just take out another sheet pan and divide the contents equally-ish between them. Nestle your slices of feta in between the other ingredients on the sheet pan, and drizzle those with a little more olive oil.

3. Pop the sheet pan into the oven, and set a timer for 30 minutes. Go about your life. When the timer goes off, check the sheet pan. You want the cherry tomatoes to have burst and to maybe have a little char on the outside, and the gnocchi to be getting golden. If they're not, bump up the heat to 450°F and give them another 5 to 10 minutes. It's OK if a few gnocchi or tomatoes come out blacker than the others, those will just be extra crunchy. Once they're at the right level of cooked, pull the pan out of the oven. Take a bite to taste for seasoning, and add more salt and pepper if you want. If using, scatter spinach or arugula over the top of the pan and mix it into the gnocchi-tomato-shallot mess. Ladle into a bowl or eat right off the sheet pan.

I Love You, Frozen Dumplings

I graduated from college in 2008, which meant that I emerged blinking into the working world just as it was plunged headfirst into a recession. I managed to find an internship that paid $10 an hour, and therefore pay my share of the rent on an apartment in Queens, but I was pretty broke for a while there, not an uncommon situation for a person in their early twenties. The food that was maybe most responsible for keeping me fed and relatively hale was dumplings. I could walk from my internship to the edge of Chinatown and get six of them for a dollar, doused in sriracha and soy sauce. I would also pick up industrial-size bags of frozen dumplings that I could bring home and cook later for dinners or post-bar snacks. Between fresh dumplings, frozen dumplings, and a lot of chickpeas, I was able to feed myself well while still allocating some of my budget for terrible cheap drinks with my friends.

Dumplings are gorgeous, glorious things, both filling and reasonably nutritious, as well as very inexpensive. I still keep a bag or two in my freezer for dinner for easy meals, though now they're usually from Trader Joe's or H Mart. They're a great way to have something quick on the table when other options feel too daunting. There are lots of ways to prepare dumplings—boiling or steaming is a classic, but you can also use them like a protein element in a larger dish and get a little bit weird with it. Here's how.

PAN-FRY THEM, THEN ADD SOME EGGS

The fry-steam-fry technique that I use for frozen ravioli and eggs comes from preparing potstickers, so it's not surprising that it's my go-to way of cooking dumplings. Don't worry about defrosting them, either. All you do is add a slick of oil to cover the bottom of a skillet that has a lid—I use canola or another neutral oil because I don't love how olive oil tastes with dumplings, but you do you—and heat it up for a minute or 2 on medium-high. Then put your dumplings into the skillet in an even layer and let them fry for a couple minutes until the bottoms of the dumplings start getting crispy and brown. Pour about ¼ cup of water into the skillet—you can eyeball it—and clap the lid onto the pan, to trap all the steam that'll cook the dumplings through. Leave that to work for another 4 or 5 minutes, until the dumplings seem cooked through and no longer frozen. It might take longer depending on the kind of dumpling you have and how big they are—that's fine, let them steam. (If the steam evaporates too soon, just add another 2 tablespoons of water.) Then lift the lid off the pan. You want all the water to evaporate so that the bottoms of the dumplings get crisp rather than soggy, which shouldn't take more than an extra minute.

At this point, if you want, you can just be done with cooking dumplings—slide them off the pan, and eat them with a dipping sauce. But if you want some extra protein in there, or just a twist on the classic, crack 2 eggs into a bowl and mix them up with a fork, just until the yolk and white are integrated. Then pour the eggs into the pan with the dumplings and attempt to swirl the pan so that the egg mixture seeps in between the dumplings. It's a thin layer, so it shouldn't take more than 2 or 3 minutes for the eggs to cook through—then flip the whole egg-dumpling pancake onto a plate. Voilà—dumpling omelet.

MAKE SOME EASY DUMPLING SAUCES

Any good platter of dumplings needs some sauces to dunk those pleasing little pockets into, and you probably already have a range of options in your condiment drawer. The classic dumpling sauce, like one you get from your local Chinese American takeout joint, is usually made of soy sauce, Chianking vinegar (sometimes just called Chinese black vinegar), and sesame oil. I don't always have Chianking vinegar handy, so I substitute rice vinegar or apple cider vinegar. I use a tablespoon of soy sauce, a tablespoon of vinegar, and a dash or 2 of sesame oil. You can adjust the ratio to your liking, and add a dash of hot sauce, chili oil, or red pepper flakes in there, as well. Another classic dumpling sauce? Mix together a tablespoon or 2 of mayonnaise and a couple heaping spoonfuls of chili crisp. If you don't have chili crisp, sriracha also works. I also like to mix sambal oelek in soy sauce as a dipping sauce, or sometimes I mix together hoisin sauce and a little bit of peanut butter.

AIR-FRY THEM, BAKE THEM, OR PUT THEM IN THE TOASTER OVEN

If you want super-crispy dumplings but don't want to deal with a pan, then behold—use your air fryer. Toss the frozen dumplings in oil and spread them evenly in an air fryer basket. Then set the air fryer to 375°F and fry the dumplings for 6 minutes. Flip them, and cook for another 2 to 4 minutes, until they're as crispy as you want them.

You can also do this in the regular oven. Set the oven to 375°F, take out a baking sheet, toss the dumplings in oil or spray them with cooking oil, and arrange them on the baking sheet so that they're not touching. (Touching reduces crisping, but if you don't mind that, it doesn't matter.) Then slide them into the oven. Take them out after 10 minutes and shake them around a bit, to unstick them from the sheet pan and expose another side of the dumpling to the hot pan for crisping, and then slide them back in for another 5 to 8 minutes.

Can you do this in a toaster oven, too? Yep, you sure can. Same rules apply as in the oven, only you can't fit quite as many dumplings on a toaster sheet as on a standard sheet pan. That's fine, if you're still hungry you can make another batch. Toss them in oil and arrange them on your toaster sheet pan, and put them in at 375°F. Check them after 8 minutes, toss them around a bit, and put them in for another 5 to 7 minutes until they're as crispy as you want.

TREAT THEM LIKE PASTA

You can treat ravioli like little dumplings, but can you treat dumplings like large-format ravioli? Friend, you sure can. That means not only can you simmer them and strain them like you would pasta, you can also sauce dumplings like you would pasta. Potstickers tossed in a tomato sauce with a hefty sprinkling of parmesan or pecorino on them are delicious. You can also toss dumplings in pesto and olive oil, or dress them in browned butter, or throw them into an Alfredo or vodka sauce. Most dumplings aren't super spiced on the inside, which means that they're essentially little pockets of meat and vegetables, like tortellini and ravioli, and so they work perfectly in many pasta recipes. (*New York Times* cooking editor Eric Kim's excellent gochujang noodle sauce—¼ cup each of gochujang, honey, and rice vinegar simmered together until it coats the back of a spatula—is incredible on dumplings, for example.) You can even put them in a casserole dish and cover them with tomato sauce and shredded mozzarella, for a kind of dumpling parmigiana. You can also just melt together a couple tablespoons of butter and a tablespoon of white miso for a salty-fatty sauce that works equally well on dumplings as it does on pasta.

BOIL THEM WITH INSTANT NOODLES AND FROZEN VEGETABLES

Here's a really easy way to bulk up frozen dumplings into a meal. Get a pot of water boiling on your stove—one that you'd usually use for pasta. Rustle up half a bag of frozen vegetables—I usually use broccoli or cauliflower, because that's what I like, but basically any frozen vegetable that you like works here. Put the frozen dumplings—as many as you want—into the pot of boiling water, add the frozen vegetables, and boil them together for 5 minutes. Then add a packet of instant noodles (like ramen noodles). Let that boil for another 2 minutes, then strain the whole thing. Toss with soy sauce and butter and voilà—an easy meal that has both protein and vegetables. If you want a little extra protein to make it more filling, just fry (or microwave!) an egg and slide it on top. Done and done.

CHOP THEM UP

If you think about dumplings as a protein source, then you can start getting into wackier territory. Could you top leftover pizza with dumplings? You could! Could you chop them up and make them into fried rice? Why not! Could you drop them into a simmering pot of soup for some extra fun soup hybrids? Why yes, you absolutely can. One of my favorite ways to use dumplings, particularly ones that I've cooked through already but are lingering leftovers in my fridge, is to chop them up into a salad. I reheat them and throw them into a pile of greens, and usually do a simple dressing, like balsamic vinegar and oil, or ginger dressing, if I have some on hand. Throw in a handful of cooked edamame and whatever vegetables you have that taste good raw, and you have a very satisfying mixing bowl salad.

MAKE A DUMPLING QUESADILLA

Remember before when I was telling you that all kinds of things are great in a quesadilla? Leftover cooked dumplings are definitely one of those. Smash your dumplings up with a fork and distribute them in a layer over a quesadilla, and top with a handful of shredded cheese, like monterey jack or cheddar. Then put another tortilla on top, warm a small amount of oil in a pan, and fry the quesadilla on both sides until the cheese is melted and the outside of the quesadilla is crispy and brown.

Stir-Fry Guy

Using a wok well is a whole art form, one I respect tremendously and am a rank amateur in. There are whole, incredible, absorbing volumes on how to make traditional stir-fried dishes. I particularly love Fuchsia Dunlop's *The Food of Sichuan* and the Leung family's *The Woks of Life*, if you want to get into the finer points of coaxing out flavor while using a wok, or learn the delights of Sichuan-style stir-fry.

But you don't need to be a master of Chinese or Chinese American cookery to make a great, satisfying stir-fry. I love a stir-fry because once you assemble the ingredients, the total time between having a pile of raw stuff from your fridge and having a cohesive meal is blazingly quick. It's particularly nice during the summer, when I want to minimize time standing over a stove, or when I have energy to cook but not for it to be a whole drawn-out process. It's also a way that I lure myself away from the siren call of too much takeout, because I can usually approximate the dish I would be ordering from my beloved Chinese takeout joint and feel virtuous for saving money and adding in more vegetables. And then when I do inevitably give in to the pull of professionally made General Tso's or mapo tofu brought directly to my door, it feels like a real treat.

STIR-FRY TOOLS AND SUPPLIES

Making an easy stir-fry is one of the things that I taught my little brother when he was in medical school and largely subsisting off of energy drinks and protein bars—you can keep a few bags of mixed frozen stir-fry vegetables and some tofu in the freezer, have a bottle of soy sauce in the pantry, and pretty much always have what you need to stir-fry on hand. You don't even need a wok, although if you love stir-frying, buying a wok is a good, relatively inexpensive addition to your kitchen. All you need is a big skillet, some oil, and some stir-frying ingredients.

The main thing you need to know going into stir-frying is that it all comes together really fast, so it's not the kind of meal that you can start cooking right away and prep as you go. You'll want to have all your vegetables and meat ready to throw into the pan before you start. You'll also want to have a bowl or plate on hand so you can dump out the ingredients from the wok or pan and add them back in at the end.

I don't know your life or your produce preferences, but if you have no idea where to start with stir-frying, those bags of frozen mixed stir-fry vegetables are a good, low-effort place. If you want to use fresh vegetables, ones that work well for stir-frying include broccoli, cauliflower, green beans, water chestnuts, baby corn, bok choy, edamame, cabbage, bean sprouts, scallions, bell peppers, mushrooms, and snow peas. Choose a couple and slice them up—another trick of stir-fry is that because everything goes in a very hot wok for a short amount of time, you need smaller pieces for them to cook through. The protein you choose should also be cut into small chunks or sliced thinly. Sliced chicken breast, ground meat, sliced sausage, cubes of tofu, and thinly sliced steak work well here.

Don't feel like you need to have a ton of stuff to make a good stir-fry. Just one or two vegetables, a meat, and a sauce work great. One of my go-to stir-frys, adapted from a recipe for string beans with pork, ginger, and red chili from Julia Turshen's book *Small Victories*, is just what it sounds like—green beans with ground pork. Beef and broccoli is also a classic pairing for a reason. You don't need a whole host of ingredients for a stir-fry to be good—in fact, the less you crowd the skillet, the crispier things will get.

STIR-FRY PLAY-BY-PLAY

Line up your chosen sliced-up ingredients and heat a wok or the largest skillet you have—if you have a choice, go with cast-iron or stainless steel and avoid nonstick—over high heat. Let the wok get really, really hot—not smoking, but it should be hot enough that if you flick some water on its surface, the water sizzles off quickly. Add 2 tablespoons of neutral oil, such as vegetable, canola, or peanut oil, and your fresh vegetables. It'll all crackle madly, and that's OK. Sauté the vegetables, stirring occasionally, until they're cooked through and charred in spots.

If you're using frozen vegetables, be extra careful about adding them to the hot pan. I usually add them to the pan without oil so they can defrost and the excess liquid can sizzle away, and then add oil after. Otherwise, the oil can spatter and burn you, which is unpleasant at best and ends in a visit to urgent care at worst. You can also defrost and drain the vegetables before adding them to the wok, which will also avoid the oil splatter problem.

Once the vegetables are cooked through—spear one with a fork and take a careful bite to make sure it's where you want it—dump them out of the wok into your waiting bowl and put the wok back over the heat.

Then add your meat or tofu and a tablespoon or 2 more neutral oil. Cook, again stirring occasionally, and add more oil if the pan seems dry. At this point, you can add minced garlic or ginger if you have it and want it. I usually add a dollop of ginger-garlic paste that I get from my local Indian grocery store, which works a treat and means I avoid mincing garlic entirely, but you can skip it. Once the protein is cooked through, add the vegetables back into the skillet.

At this point, your stir-fry is cooked, but you probably want to add some kind of sauce or seasoning to bring it all together. Because in stir-fry you generally want to avoid extra liquid—and adding salt to vegetables has the effect of drawing out liquid—I wait until the end to add a sauce instead of seasoning or salting the ingredients while cooking. The simplest stir-fry sauce I know is 2 tablespoons of soy sauce and 2 tablespoons of white wine or chicken stock, mixed together. Drizzle it over the hot ingredients while they're still in the wok (you can turn the stove off first) and stir it into the stir-fry. A dash of sriracha, chili oil, or sambal oelek would work well here, or any of the packaged stir-fry sauces you can usually find in the grocery

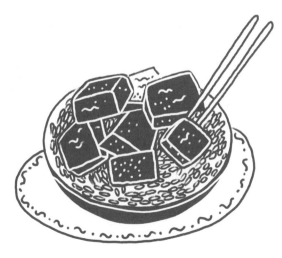

store. You can also dissolve about a tablespoon of brown sugar and a teaspoon or 2 of hot sauce into ¼ cup of soy sauce and use that as an excellent stir-fry sauce, one I adapted from Beth Moncel, who runs the website Budget Bytes. She uses it for her great, easy dragon noodles, a recipe that has prevented me from shrugging and ordering takeout on multiple occasions.

Use some kitchen shears to snip scallions over the top of the stir-fry if you want, or you can finish it with a sprinkling of sesame seeds. Or you can skip all that, throw it into a bowl, and eat it. I usually eat my stir-fry over rice or instant noodles, but there's no law that says you need to.

Do Curry, Be Happy

The word *curry* is sort of like the word *gravy*, in that it can refer to a vast number of dishes of various complexities and origins. You could be talking about a Thai red curry with tender beef and squash, or a Bengali-style doi murgi, or a Sri Lankan parippu, or a Goan vindaloo, or the curry powder mayonnaise dipping sauce that comes alongside french fries in an Irish fish and chips spot. You can recreate any of those at home if you want, but you don't need to feel harnessed to any particular culinary tradition to recognize that curry is delicious, and using curry powder or curry paste is a quick, easy way to get a lot of flavor into a dish that would otherwise be lackluster.

Usually when I make a curry or curry-ish meal in my house, it has Indian influences. I spent a couple months in Mumbai as a naive but enthusiastic college student and fell completely in love with South Indian food, so making my own weird approximations of dal and saag paneer is a particular comfort to me. If you have the interest and wherewithal to do some exploring of Indian and Indian American cuisine, I swear by Madhur Jaffrey's many excellent books, and I'd also point you to the fantastic *Indian-ish* by Priya Krishna and *Amrikan* by Khushbu Shah, my brilliant buddy who opened my eyes to the delights of yogurt rice. But again, you don't need to worry about any of that to deploy curry in a way that'll get you a meal quickly and deliciously.

CURRY IN A HURRY

Curry powder or paste is one of my go-to spice mixes for adding a little bit of zazz to anything I'm eating. (You can find curry paste in the international aisle in many grocery stores—generally some with the Thai ingredients and some with the Indian, depending on curry type—but if you don't have that kind of grocery store you can order it online.) When I'm roasting a sheet pan of vegetables, for example, sometimes I toss in a tablespoon or so of curry powder along with oil, salt, and pepper to coat the vegetables. You can stir some into your soup or beans to give it a little extra something. It's also a nice way to add flavor to a plain piece of meat, like a chicken breast or thigh or a salmon filet.

But one of my favorite tricks is just stirring in a tablespoon (or a few, depending on how much spice I want) of curry powder or paste into coconut milk, simmering some vegetables and whatever protein I have around in it—rotisserie chicken, some cut-up tofu, a can of beans—until it cooks down a little, ladling it over rice and calling it a curry. You can also keep cooking the curry-paste-and-coconut-milk mixture down until it's more of a glazy sauce if you prefer. Nutrition, flavor, done.

That principle is how I came up with this approximation of the absolutely stellar Northern Thai dish khao soi, which is a curry soup with soft noodles cooked into the curry and crunchy noodles on top, plus some kind of meat, like bone-in chicken, topped with mustard greens and various herbs. It's great, and making it from scratch would take forever, and require a lot of chopping. But thanks to the beauty of premade curry paste or powder, plus instant noodles, I figured out a kind of dirtbag vegetarian version of khao soi that involves frozen vegetables, chickpeas, and basically no time to make. The curry base is inspired by Budget Bytes's Beth Moncel's coconut curry ramen, and the rest is inspired by having no time or willpower to do anything except empty things into a pot.

Do Exactly This: Sort-of Khao Soi

This is a recipe that's absolutely meant to be messed with—add what sounds delicious to you, omit the noodles and serve it over rice, substitute meat for the chickpeas, use fresh vegetables if you have them, simmer some garlic and ginger with the curry powder. Put a handful of quick cooking greens, like kale or spinach, in with the instant noodles. Throw cilantro on top at the end. Whatever you want to do. Think about it as a loosely sketched road map I gave you on a bar napkin that you can fill in however you want.

Ingredients

- 1 tablespoon neutral oil, like canola
- 2 tablespoons curry powder or curry paste (Thai red or massaman curry paste works great here, but anything you have on hand will work, and feel free to increase or decrease this amount based on your spice

tolerance)
- *1 15.5-ounce can chickpeas, drained*
- *1 12- or 16-ounce bag frozen vegetables*
- *1 13.5-ounce can coconut milk*
- *2 packets instant ramen noodles*
- *Salt and pepper*

Optional
- *½ teaspoon red pepper flakes*

1. Get out a medium or large pot, one that you could cook spaghetti in. Put it on the stove over medium heat, and add the neutral oil. Wait about a minute for it to get hot, and then add curry powder or paste and red pepper flakes, if you're using them.

2. Use a spatula to stir the powder or paste into the oil and cook it until it starts smelling like curry, usually about 30 seconds to a minute. Then add your chickpeas and vegetables, and stir until the curry oil is incorporated into the chickpea-vegetable mix. Don't worry about it evenly coating everything; the idea is just to distribute it a little bit.

3. Dump in your can of coconut milk. Then fill the can up with water, and dump that in too. It's fine if the vegetables aren't totally submerged—they'll still defrost and cook. Raise the heat to high until the mixture boils, then turn it down until it's simmering. Add 1½ bricks of ramen noodles, and bring it back up to a simmer. Cook for 2 minutes—take a vegetable out of the pot and carefully take a bite to make sure it's

cooked all the way through. If not, give it another minute or 2 of simmering until it gets there. Taste the sauce. Add salt and pepper, and taste again. Repeat until it tastes good to you.

4. Scoop the curry into bowls. Grab the remaining half brick of ramen noodles and crumble some of it over the bowls, as a garnish.

You're Telling Me a Shrimp Fried This Rice?

It is always a minor cause for celebration in my house when there's leftover rice, whether from a takeout order or from just making too much of the stuff, because that means the next day I can cosplay as a cook at Benihana and make fried rice. You can use fresh rice to make fried rice if you want—just spread it out on a sheet pan and let it dry out a little. But rice that has dried out a bit in the refrigerator works best for fried rice because a lot of the moisture has already evaporated from its surface, meaning that it can crisp up a lot more easily in a pan.

There are all kinds of schools of thought about fried rice and its various components. You can use a lot of sauce or just a little, incorporate a ton of vegetables or just a sprinkling, use oil or butter, use fresh chilled rice or the stale leftover kind. All of these are valid—really, whatever you decide you prefer is the correct way to make it. What matters for us is that fried rice is super easy and even better when it's made out of leftovers. Everything else is details.

FRIED RICE FUNDAMENTALS

To make basic fried rice, what you need is neutral oil, soy sauce, left-over rice (2 cups is ideal but use however much you have), and 1 or 2 eggs. To make things easier as you're working with the skillet, it's worth going ahead and cracking the eggs into a little bowl and whisking them up so that there's no distinct yolk or white. Things that are nice to add if you have them: sliced-up green onions (use your shears for this), a cup of frozen or precooked vegetables (those bags of frozen peas, carrots, and corn kernels are a go-to for me, or a stir-fry mix), oyster sauce, chili oil or sriracha, and sesame oil. If you have cooked meat, like shredded rotisserie chicken or leftover cooked ground meat, that's a great add-in. Quick-cooking seafood, like shrimp, is also fantastic in fried rice. If you want more protein but not meat, cubed tofu is great—I would sear it before you throw it into the fried rice. Quick-cooking vegetables like snow peas or asparagus are great too. Just make sure that anything you add is already in bite-size pieces, since they won't be spending enough time in the pan to cook, just enough to warm through.

You want to break out your largest skillet, something that gives you a lot of room to stir things around without risk of the ingredients overflowing the edges. If you have a wok, even better, use that. Put your wok or skillet over high heat and let it get very hot. Then add 2 tablespoons of neutral oil and swirl it around so it coats the skillet. You want the oil to be hot, but not so hot that it starts smoking—no fire hazards if we can help it.

Drop the rice into the skillet, then break up any clumps with a wooden spoon. If you like having little toasted, golden patches of rice, the trick here is to let the rice hang out in the skillet and fry for a few minutes before you start stirring it around. If not, start stirring right away. The idea is to get every single grain of rice coated with a little oil, but you know, do your best, no one is taking a microscope to your fried rice.

Make a little hole in the middle of the rice by scooting the rice toward the sides of the skillet or wok with the wooden spoon. If the pan looks dry, pour another tablespoon of oil into the bare patch. Then add your egg, leaving it to cook for about a minute. Once the egg starts setting, scramble it with your wooden spoon, and then mix the scrambled pieces into the rice, tossing the mixture around.

If you have frozen or quick-cooking vegetables, cooked protein, or green onions to add to the rice, now's the time to add them. Repeat the process of making a bare spot in the bottom of the pan by piling the rice toward the sides, and add the protein or vegetables into the bare spot. Leave them for a minute or two to develop a little bit of char on the edges, and to get a chance to thaw out if they're frozen. Then mix them into the rice and egg. Turn off the heat.

SEASON AND SAUCE

Now comes the fun part: seasoning the fried rice. For a simple seasoning, just add a tablespoon of soy sauce and mix it so it's evenly distributed throughout the fried rice. But you don't have to stop there. A glug of oyster sauce or hoisin sauce is lovely here, and a teaspoon or more of chili oil or hot sauce works great too. If you have sesame oil, mixing in a dash or two into the rice will give it a lovely nutty flavor. The easy stir-fry sauce that I wrote about earlier—soy sauce, brown sugar, sriracha—is also great.

There's controversy in the fried rice community about how much sauce to use—after putting in the work to get the rice all crispy, do you really want to drown it in sauce? But I say do whatever makes you happy. Add a little or a lot. Soy sauce is usually fairly salty, but it's still worth tasting the rice to see if it needs more salt—after all it's just a big pile of grains, and those usually need seasoning. I like to add a lot of black pepper to pretty much anything I cook, and fried rice is no exception, but you could skip it in favor of chili crisp or red pepper flakes if you want a little more of a kick. If you like teppanyaki-style fried rice, swap out some of the neutral oil for unsalted butter, which will give you that unctuous note. I like to top my fried rice with fried shallots from giant bags of the stuff I pick up at H Mart or fried garlic chips for a little extra crunch. If you happen to have any leftover fried wonton strips knocking around—like the kind that come with egg-drop soup—those are incredible on top of a batch of fried rice.

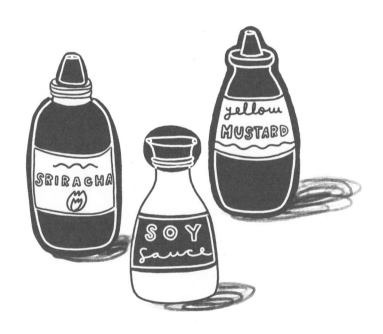

The Cooking Treat

We all know you have earned a little treat if you, say, finish something at work, or start something at work, or do your laundry, or think hard about doing your laundry. Cooking is no different. If it's hard to convince yourself to see your casserole ambitions through, may I suggest a cooking treat?

The classic cooking treat is a glass of the same wine you're cooking with, but it doesn't have to be alcoholic—I personally love a giant glass of extremely bubbly seltzer as I'm working. And it doesn't have to be a beverage at all. If you're cooking and there's a delicious scrap, that little bit is all yours. If you're baking, the treat is almost always getting to lick the spoon (yes I know about salmonella). But no cookie dough or icing need be involved for you to get a little snack bonus. Maybe you reserve a hunk of the feta that you're crumbling to eat with crackers. Maybe as you're cutting up your vegetables you cut up an extra pepper that you can dunk into ranch dressing and snack on as you go. The knife and cutting board are already out, so you may as well, right? Or go for a handful of granola or a helping of chocolate chips, since you're already standing near the cabinets. Whatever you snack on, you earned it.

Casseroles Are Anarchists

A casserole is the gift that keeps on giving. There's a reason that it's *the* go-to dish for dropping off at people's doorsteps during times of transition—new baby, new house, death in the family, illness, bad news, good news, medium news. A casserole can accommodate seemingly every human feeling, and pretty darn close to every human food. It's an inherently generous dish. No matter what kind it is, a casserole—or hotdish if you're Minnesotan—promises comfort, the ease of a home-cooked meal that you don't have to put any thought into. This is probably the heaviest lift, cooking-wise, in this book, because it involves cooking a few components and then adding them to another dish that you have to cook once *again*, so if it's too much, skip it. But if it intrigues you—and the idea of having sustaining leftovers for the week (or beyond, if you freeze it) is enticing—then read on. If you invest energy into putting together a casserole, that casserole will pay it back in dividends.

WHAT EVEN IS A CASSEROLE?

In many ways, a casserole is an amalgam of all the other foods in this book. It's kind of like a dip but with a starch mixed in, or maybe it's more like a solid stew, or a non-eggy frittata, or even *very* chonky nachos. Or maybe it's none of those—you get to decide. The point is, the category of casserole can expand to include nearly anything your heart desires. You can have cheeseburger casserole, but also a three-bean casserole, tikka masala casserole, french onion casserole, lamb casserole that has feta and crumbled pita chips on top, or egg roll casserole that has pork, cabbage, and spring onions topped with crunchy wontons. Those all count. I once went on a day-long internet dive trying to figure out what exactly defines a casserole, and the best answer that I could find is that it's named after the kind of dish it's served in. Obviously that's bonkers—if I serve you a pile of celery in a pie dish that doesn't make it celery pie—but it points to just how thoroughly casseroles acknowledge neither gods nor masters. Casseroles are beautiful, edible anarchy contained in a dish. Is a lasagna technically a casserole? That's not a question I can answer, but signs point to maybe.

How does that help you, exactly? A couple ways. First, if you have more people to feed on a daily basis, a casserole is an easy way to accomplish that without a lot of fuss or forethought. Second, you can treat yourself like a neighbor in a sitcom—if you know you're going to have a tough time ahead but you have a little extra energy now, making a casserole and eating it throughout the week is a godsend. You can also freeze part or all of it for later and reap those dividends when you're at a low point.

All casseroles follow a basic formula, and it's easy enough to figure out. Measurements in casseroles are loose, so don't stress if you're a little bit over or under any of these things. Here is my Universal Casserole Formula. For a casserole of any kind, you need:

2 cups of vegetables: These can be fresh, frozen, or canned. Green beans are a classic, but any vegetable that stands up to cooking would work—broccoli, cauliflower, cubed squash, black beans, chickpeas, canned green chilis, diced onion, bell peppers, mushrooms, frozen corn, frozen peas, spinach, you name it. Just leave out tender lettuces; keep those for a side salad.

2 cups of cooked meat, or meat-like thing: We're talking ground beef, turkey, pork, chicken, lamb, or your favorite meatless substitute (I really like soy chorizo in a casserole). Canned tuna is a classic.

Shredded rotisserie chicken once again comes in handy. Lentils or beans would work if you want to keep it vegetarian. Sausage is a great ingredient for casserole because it's basically just heavily seasoned ground meat—you can take it out of the casing, cook it through, set it aside, and be done. Chopped-up dumplings would work! Leftover ham from the holiday party, cubed up. Whatever you've got that needs using. Just be sure to cook the protein all the way through if it isn't cooked already.

2 cups of cooked starchy things: By this I mean rice, noodles, or another cooked grain such as quinoa or farro. Shredded or cut-up raw potatoes work here, too, and in fact frozen hash browns are pretty excellent in a casserole. Also? Tater tots or other frozen potato products are great—you can layer them on the top of a casserole so that they crisp up and give the whole thing structure.

1 to 2 cups of a binder: Casseroles need a binder to impart some extra flavor and bring the whole mess together. Sure, you can make a béchamel if that's something you have time and energy for, but traditionally the casserole saucing comes from a can or jar. You can use tomato sauce, vodka sauce, vegetable or chicken broth, gravy, a jar of salsa, or a canned, thick condensed soup such as cream of mushroom or cream of chicken. A combination of any of these counts as a binder. Sour cream works, too, or if all else fails, just crack 3 eggs into a bowl, whisk them together, and call it a day.

1 to 2 cups of cheese (optional, but take the option): Not every casserole *needs* cheese, but it's rare that you find a casserole that won't be improved by cheese. Use the bagged, shredded kind here, no need to deplete your fancy cheese stores. Shredded cheddar, monterey jack, mozzarella, and parmesan are all lovely. Crumbled feta will yield delicious little salty pockets in the casserole.

1 cup of topping: This, too, is optional, but I wouldn't skip it. One of the best parts of a casserole is the crunchy topping, contrasting with the delightful amalgamated mush underneath. And this topping, boy, it can really be *anything.* Crumbled-up chips of all sorts make excellent casserole topping. Butter crackers or saltines, crunched up, absolutely. Cheez-Its or crumbled-up Goldfish crackers add cheesiness and also whimsy. Really, any savory cracker will work. You can also use cereal, like Chex or cornflakes, as long as it's not sweet. (Lucky Charms casserole intrigues me conceptually but I think it would be a little hideous to eat.) Canned fried onions or fried shallots are incredible on top of a casserole. Plain old breadcrumbs work fine, too, if that's what you have knocking around. Assess your salty snacks and you'll almost certainly find something.

Seasoning: Basic salt and pepper work just fine in a casserole, but you can also throw in any of the seasoning mixes that I touched on before. Taco seasoning, curry powder, garam masala, berbere, powdered harissa, whatever's on hand.

MAKE YOUR CASSEROLE

Remember, all your meats have to be cooked already, so do that if you need to. Get out a 9-by-13-inch dish and set your oven to 350°F. Don't have a casserole dish? Use a cast-iron skillet. Don't have a cast-iron skillet? Use whatever oven-safe pan you have—cake pan, brownie pan, whatever. To the dish add all the ingredients except for the topping, and stir it around. Once it seems pretty homogenous, sprinkle your chosen topping over the casserole surface, aiming to get in a layer that covers the whole thing. Cover the dish with aluminum foil. Bake for 30 minutes. Take the foil off and check in—are the edges bubbling? Is the topping browned enough to your liking? If so, pull it out. If not, give it another 5 to 10 minutes. Done.

If all that seems sort of helpful but you need an actual, real world example of a casserole that works, you can follow the specific recipe on page 173. The origins of this one are simple. I was at my best friend Katie's lake house in Alabama one Fourth of July, and woke up the next morning with a variety of party leftovers and a dream: to convert those into a casserole. After consulting by text message at length with my personal casserole thought leader (and fancy food writer) Kat Kinsman, we came up with what is affectionately known as Dirtbag Lakehouse Casserole. It's delicious, and easy enough to make when you are mildly hungover and need to eat something.

Following is a riff on that recipe, which will henceforth be known as Party Leftovers Casserole. Technically it does not contain vegetables, unless you consider tater tots to be a vegetable, but I think it's a good example of just how easy and accommodating a casserole can be—once you've Done Exactly This once or twice, you'll have a good foundation for swapping out elements in your casserole to accommodate what you have on hand. Don't have sausage but have ground turkey? OK, cool! Don't have sour cream, but have a can of cream of mushroom soup? Love that for you. No tater tots in sight but you have those smiley face potato rounds, frozen hash browns, or frozen french fries? Right on, it'll work. I've made this with Bagel Bites instead of tater tots, mozzarella instead of Mexican cheese, and an assortment of grab-bag stale spices that I rustled up instead of taco blend. I use whatever bottom-of-the-bag chips are hanging out, including Tostitos, sour cream and onion kettle chips, Takis, and Cool Ranch Doritos. It works perfectly. If you want to add things or subtract them, by all means: it's your party.

Do Exactly This: Party Leftovers Casserole

This is a riff on a casserole I've made a couple times to sustain people during various vacations where an amount of Bud Light was likely consumed. It is still good even if you aren't hungover, which is the true test of a casserole. It is also extremely flexible. You can use a vast array of party leftovers, as long as they aren't, like, a sushi tray or a soup tasting course. (But if you have these at your parties, please do invite me.)

Ingredients

- 14 to 16 ounces crumbled breakfast sausage (real or fake meat)
- 3 eggs
- 1 cup milk (I like whole, but any, including plant based, will work)
- 2 tablespoons taco seasoning
- Salt and pepper
- 1 32-ounce bag tater tots (you'll probably have leftovers and that is fine!)
- 2 cups shredded Mexican cheese blend, or other shredded cheese
- 1 cup crushed nacho cheese Doritos, or whatever crumbled-up chips you have around

1. Turn your oven on to 350°F. Grab a 9-by-13-inch casserole

dish—it's the same size that you might make brownies in. If you have a pan that's slightly smaller or larger, that'll work too, but if it's smaller you'll want to cook the casserole for about 5 extra minutes. If it's bigger, check on the casserole 5 minutes earlier than the time recommended below.

2. Grab a skillet or frying pan. Put the sausage into the cold pan and place it on the stove over medium heat—starting in a cold pan helps render out that delicious sausage fat. Cook, breaking up the sausage with a spatula or wooden spoon, until no pink bits remain and the outside of the sausage starts to brown. This usually takes me about 5 to 7 minutes, but your mileage may vary.

3. Once the sausage is cooked through, dump it into the casserole dish. In a medium-size bowl, whisk together the eggs and the milk, and add the taco seasoning as well. Add a few shakes or cranks of pepper and a little salt—since sausage is generally salty, and you'll have the cheese going in too, go easy on the salt here. Stir it all together, and then add the mixture to the casserole dish and stir to incorporate the sausage.

4. To the top of the sausage-egg mixture, layer on your frozen tater tots. You want them to cover the top of the casserole completely but not overlap. Then sprinkle the shredded cheese blend on top of the tots, and on top of that, add a layer of crushed chips. Don't worry about it being perfectly evenly distributed—this is a casserole, not a rocket.

5. Cover the casserole dish in tin foil and stick it in the oven to bake for 30 minutes. When the timer goes off, unwrap it and

assess the situation. Is the cheese on top melted? Is it bubbling at the corners? Does the top look browned and crispy? If so, you're done. If not, add another 5 minutes to get things where you need them. (This can take up to 45 minutes depending on your oven and the stubbornness of your tater tots.) Pull the casserole out and let it cool for about 10 minutes. Then scoop it out and serve on plates or in bowls. It'll keep in the fridge for a week.

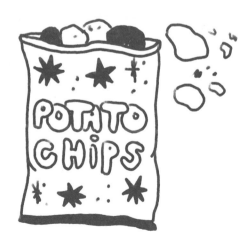

Roll Your Own Casserole

Are you ready to be your own meal train, making some casseroles to freeze for a rainy day, but you're not sure where to start? Roll a die to guide you to a cooked protein, a starch, a binder, a vegetable, a topping, and a cheese, and pop that in the oven.

COOKED PROTEIN

1. Ground meat or meat substitute
2. Meatballs
3. Sausage
4. Beans
5. Canned tuna
6. Shredded chicken

STARCH

1. Tater tots
2. Egg noodles
3. Ramen
4. Brown rice
5. White rice
6. Frozen shredded hash browns

BINDER

1. Cream of mushroom, celery, or chicken soup
2. Two eggs scrambled into one cup milk
3. Chicken or vegetable stock
4. Sour cream
5. Tomato sauce
6. Gravy

FRESH OR FROZEN VEGETABLES

1. Peas
2. Broccoli
3. Cauliflower
4. Mushrooms
5. Spinach
6. Onion

TOPPINGS

1. Fried onions
2. Potato chips
3. Breadcrumbs
4. Tortilla chips
5. Cracker crumbs
6. Unsweetened cornflakes

CHEESE

1. Mozzarella
2. Cheddar
3. Pepper jack
4. Gouda
5. American
6. "Mexican" or "taco" blend

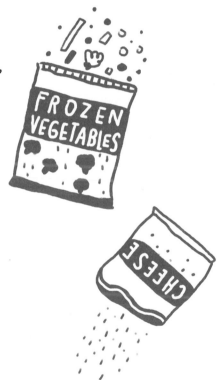

Help, I Need Dessert

In the Eby family, no dinner is complete without a little something sweet at the end. Usually, because my dad is a baking whiz, that's some delightful little pastry. But I did not inherit his love of making double crust pies as a relaxing activity. Sure, I can get into a complicated baking project on occasion, but if I have limited energy, I'm focusing on the meal part of the meal. Dessert kind of goes by the wayside, particularly since a bar of chocolate or an ice cream sandwich works perfectly fine as something sweet.

But sometimes I want something in-between—a dessert that's fun and easy to put together, maybe two steps up from eating an Oreo but nothing requiring me to break out the stand mixer. And that's when I know it's time for S'mores cones.

S'mores cones are an excellent no-recipe recipe, one that harnesses the flavor of the campfire classic, but without the inevitable problem of lighting a marshmallow on fire or getting chocolate goo all over your face and hands. You can keep the ingredients on hand to assemble one basically whenever you want—it's one of my back pocket moves for when kids come over to my house. All you need is aluminum foil, sugar or waffle cones (the kind you use for ice cream), marshmallows (I like the mini kind here for more even marshmallow distribution, but the big guys work too), and chocolate chips. Fill the cone with your preferred ratio of chocolate and marshmallow, and then wrap it in aluminum foil so no bare spots of cone are showing. Stick it in the oven at 350°F for 10 minutes. You can also do this in the toaster oven if you can't deal with the big oven. Then unwrap the cone—it should have a good mixture of melted marshmallow and chocolate in there—and eat with some care (it's gooey!).

S'mores cones also work with all manner of chocolate or candy. Leftover Halloween fun-size bars, chopped up? Yep. Butterscotch or white chocolate chips? For sure. Candy corn, for some reason? I dunno, try it, why not? If you're actually camping or you have a firepit in the backyard, you can also throw the cones in the fire for about 5 minutes and then retrieve them. And if you're grilling, or invited to a barbecue where a grill will be present, you can also put these on the grill for about 5 minutes to achieve the same effect.

Conclusion

Go Eat Something

Eating is a basic need, but putting the things together to *make* something to eat—that has challenges. Figuring out simple cooking solutions to the stretches when you have to feed yourself but do not have the energy to do so will free up your limited internal resources for other, more pressing things, whether that's taking care of children (not me) or watching ten episodes of the British show *Taskmaster* in a row (me). Cooking, with all its rules and traditions and finicky parts, can be intimidating, but if I can leave you with one piece of *You Gotta Eat* wisdom it is this: there is no higher authority in your kitchen than you. You are the ultimate expert on what you like to eat, and how, and so you can't be wrong about it. You have food instincts, even if you don't cook much, borne from what you like or dislike eating. So lean into that. You are the captain of your ship. You can decide what spices work and which don't, whether that soup needs an extra tomato or not. It doesn't matter what I think, or what Martha Stewart thinks, or what any other culinary professional thinks about the technique. You made food you want to eat, or at least find tolerable? You won the game. Do not stress about what anyone else in the world has to say about your dinner. You made dinner. That is the ultimate victory.

Also remember: cooking is forgiving. If you are in the middle of cooking and things are too much—you're feeling overwhelmed and panicked—you can always turn off the stove, take a deep breath and organize yourself, and then turn the stove back on. I did this all the time in culinary school. You just mentally add a couple minutes to get the pot or pan back up to the temperature you were working with, and keep going. Cooking is flexible like that, and since you're at home, and not the line cook of a busy restaurant, you can always take a break until things feel like they're more in control.

Also? It's just a meal. It's OK! Not every meal you eat is going to be the best one ever. Sometimes you need to buy a sandwich at the airport. It is enough to feed yourself and move on. It doesn't need to be anything more complicated than that. If you find something that works for you when time is short and energy is low, do it. In a perfect world cooking would always be a source of joy and creativity. But in this world, all it needs to be is a source of food.

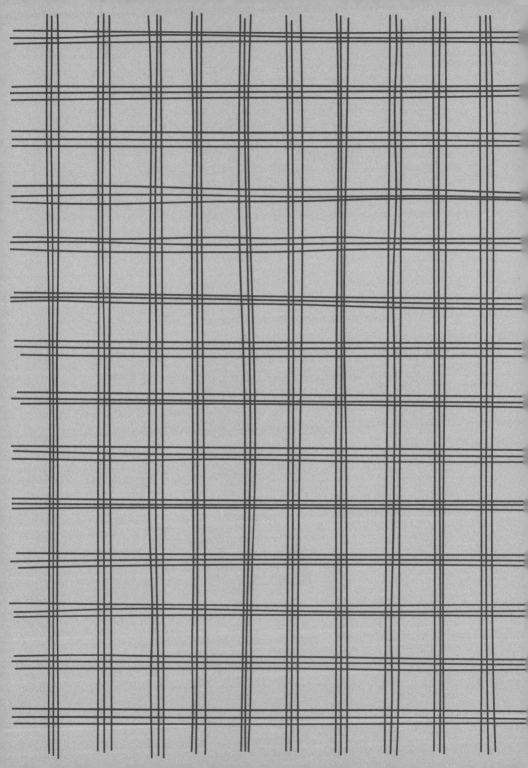

Appendix

Let's Talk About Groceries

The whole process of acquiring groceries can be fraught and exhausting. There are too many kinds of everything! Do I need this jar of salted capers? Wait, did that recipe say shallots or scallions? If the very idea of standing in an aisle perusing the different kinds of rice feels like too much for you, remember that grocery delivery exists in many places. When I'm at my most depressed, it's basically the only way that fruit exists in my home. In more rural areas of the country, you may not be able to get the groceries delivered to your door, but many grocery stores still have the option for you to shop ahead and then roll up to the store and pick up your groceries without any further interaction.

If you need some help figuring out what to pick up, I hear you, I've been there. Read on for some ideas.

ITEMS THAT LAST BASICALLY FOREVER AND CONSTITUTE A MEAL

If you just need a base layer of ingredients that you can use to make a meal when you feel like it, and you'd prefer if that stuff took a very long time to go bad, start here. Any of the ingredients below will last a long, long time tucked away in the pantry or the freezer, and if you have them on hand, you'll always be able to make yourself a meal.

- Rice
- Dried pasta (instant ramen, shelf-stable gnocchi, boxed macaroni and cheese)
- Canned beans
- Canned fish (tuna, salmon)
- Bouillon cubes or concentrate
- Oatmeal
- Pickles
- Canned or frozen vegetables
- Frozen fruit
- Frozen dumplings
- Frozen ravioli
- Olive oil (for cooking the above)

ITEMS THAT LAST BASICALLY FOREVER AND WILL MAKE THINGS TASTE BETTER

Groceries in this section will not make a meal, but they will improve a meal! Pick up anything that catches your eye—most of these will last a long time in the fridge (mayo is the fastest to go bad, but it's still a long-hauler) and will help dress up anything you make.

- Condiments of all kinds (I especially recommend the very versatile chili crisp)
- Mayonnaise
- Spice mixes (taco seasoning, curry powder, Italian seasoning, etc.)
- Vinegar (white wine, red wine, apple cider)
- Tomato paste or anchovy paste
- Salt and pepper
- Peanut butter

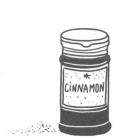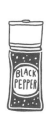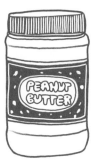

FOODS THAT LAST A MONTH OR MORE

These are good to keep on hand for adding variety and joy to the ingredients above. They last a long time (longer than you probably think, in some cases, like eggs!), so you can safely buy more if you run out, even if you don't have specific plans for what you want to make with them. They'll probably get used!

- Eggs
- Potatoes
- Onions
- Butter (you can freeze it if you need to)
- Shredded cheese

 *APPENDIX*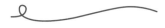

- Tortillas (these also freeze really well)
- Sliced bread (you can freeze and toast direct from freezer)

ITEMS THAT WILL MAKE YOUR LIFE EASIER

The grocery store is intimidating partly because it's full of stuff you still have to *do things to*. Instead, cut up to several steps from your food preparation routine by giving yourself permission to buy things that are already processed!

- Rotisserie chicken
- Precut fruit and vegetables
- Precut onions (a kind of vegetable, but even worse to cut up)
- Frozen fruit and vegetables
- Frozen minced garlic
- Frozen minced herbs
- Already hard-boiled eggs

Index of Recipes

anything salad sandwich, 61–62

bacon, microwaving, 64, 102
baked potatoes, 93–95
bean salad, 18–20
Black Bean Blender Soup, 120–21
BLTs, 63–64
blue cheese sauce, 122
buffalo sauce, 123

cake, 103–5
canapés, 73–75
casseroles, 168–77
cheese board, 56–61
cheese sauce, 52–53
chili, 38–44
chili dip, 68–69
cocktail sauce, sort-of, 122
cowboy caviar, 72
Crispy Gnocchi and Tomatoes, 147–49
curry, 159–63

dessert, 178–79
dessert sauce, 123
dips, 67–72; cowboy caviar, 72; The Easiest Dip I Know, 71; hummus, 112–15
dumplings, frozen, 149–55

Easiest Dip I Know, The, 71
egg in the middle, 133–34
esquites, 70

finger foods, 76–78
fried eggs, 127–28
fried rice, 163–66
frittatas, 131–33
frozen dumplings, 149–55

gnocchi, 145–49
grab-bag green sauce, 115–17
green goddess-y dressing, 122
green sauce, grab bag, 115–17

hors d'oeuvres, 76–78
hummus, 112–15

Khao Soi, Sort-of, 161–63

lasagna, ramen, 49

mac and cheese, 49–53
miso dressing, 122
Mushroom Bites, Three Ingredient, 76–78

nachos, 78–81
noodles, 142–45, 153. See also ramen

oatmeal, 91–93
olive tapenade, 69–70
omelets, 128–30

Party Leftovers Casserole, 173–75
pasta, 142–45, 153. See also ramen
popcorn, 88–91
potatoes, 93–95

quesadillas, 65–67, 154–55
queso, 68

raita, 69
ramen, 44–49
ravioli, 142–44, 153
rice in a mug, 98

salad, bean, 18–20
salad dressing, 19
salmon dip, 69
sandwiches, 21–27, 61–64
sauces, 121–23, 144–45, 151–52, 165–66
sheet pan meals, 135–39
sheet pan vegetables, sauce for, 122
smoothies, 108–11
s'mores cones, 178–79
Sort-of Khao Soi, 161–63
soup / stew, 29–36, 119–21; Black Bean Blender Soup, 120–21; Tomato Sauce Soup, 34–36
stir-fry, 155–59
stir-fry sauce, 122, 165–66

Thai-inspired sauce, 123
Three-Ingredient Mushroom Bites, 76–78
Throw-Everything-in-a-Pot Chili, 42–44
toast, 27–28
Tomato Sauce Soup, 34–36
Two-Ingredient Mug Cake, 104–5

umami sauce for grain bowls, 122

vegetables, dip for, 122

yogurt, 81–85

Index of Ingredients

anchovies, 69–70
apples, 24–25
artichoke hearts, 62–63
arugula, 85, 91, 147–49
avocado, 25

bacon, 41, 63–64, 102
bananas, 24–25
beans: bean salad, 18–20;
Black Bean Blender
Soup, 120–21; cowboy
caviar, 72; quesadillas,
66; stews, 31–32;
Throw-Everything-in-a-
Pot Chili, 43; vinegar
and brown sugar in, 41
beer, 38–39, 43
black-eyed peas, 72
blue cheese, 69
Boursin, 77
brown sugar, 41
butter, 23, 48, 96, 123

celery, 24–25
cheese: casseroles,
170–71; cheese board,
56–61; Crispy Gnocchi
and Tomatoes, 147–49;
mac and cheese, 51;
nachos, 79–81; Party
Leftovers Casserole,
173–75; quesadillas,
65–67; ramen, 45–46;
sandwiches, 24. See
also feta; parmesan;
pecorino
chickpeas, 112–15, 161–63
chips: chili, 41–42; Party
Leftovers Casserole,
173–75; sandwiches,
26–27. See also
toppings
chocolate chips, 178–79
chutney, 24
cocoa powder, 39

coconut milk, 32, 161–63
corn, 43, 70, 72
cottage cheese, 117–18
cream, 34–36
cream cheese, 26, 77
cucumber, 25
curry paste, 161–63
curry powder, 32, 161–63

dumplings, frozen,
149–55

eggs, 126–34; fried rice,
163–66; frozen
dumplings, 150–51;
microwaving, 99–101;
Party Leftovers
Casserole, 173–75;
ramen, 47
eyeballing
measurements, 14–15

feta, 25, 118, 136, 147–49,
171
frozen dumplings, 149–55
fruit, 109

gnocchi, 145–49
goat cheese, 63
green chilis, 43
groceries, buying, 183–86

half and half, 34–36
herbs, 29–30, 34–36
honey, 24
hot sauce, 24, 47
hummus, 25, 112–15

jalapeños, 40
jam, 23–24

ketchup, 51
kitchen shears, 140–41

leftovers: eggs, 101;
quesadillas, 66–67;
stews, 33–34
lentils, 32

marshmallows, 178–79
mayo, 22–23, 61–62, 70,
122, 152, 184
measurements,
eyeballing, 14–15
meat: casseroles, 169–70;
fried rice, 163–66; mac
and cheese, 52;
quesadillas, 66; sheet
pan meals, 136; stews,
33–34; stir-fry, 155–59
milk, 34–36, 173–75
miso paste, 30, 48
mushrooms, 76–78

noodles, 142–45, 153, 170.
See also ramen

oatmeal, 91–93
olive oil, 34–36, 71, 114,
137
olives, 26, 69–70

parmesan, 35–36, 48, 53,
77–78, 80
pasta, 33–34, 142–45, 153,
170. See also ramen
peanut butter, 24–25, 47
peas, 51
pecorino, 35–36, 53,
77–78
pickles, 25–26
pineapple, 22
popcorn, 88–91
potatoes, 93–95, 170,
173–75. See also tater
tots

protein: casseroles, 169–70; dumplings as, 154; fried rice, 163–66; mac and cheese, 52; quesadillas, 66; stews, 33–34; stir-fry, 155–59

ramen, 44–49; frozen dumplings, 153–54; Sort-of Khao Soi, 161–63
ravioli, 142–44, 153
rice, 98, 163–66, 170

salmon, 69
salsa, 40, 43, 120–21
sausage, 33, 136, 170, 173–75
seitan bacon, 63–64
shears, 140–41
soup toppings, 34
sour cream, 69, 71
spices, 37; casseroles, 171; chili, 39–40; mac and cheese, 50; sheet pan meals, 137–38; Throw-Everything-in-a-Pot Chili, 43
spinach, 144, 147–49
stew toppings, 34
sugar cones, 178–79
sweet toppings, 84

tahini, 114
tater tots, 58, 170, 172, 173–75
tomatoes, 22, 32, 43, 72, 147–49
tomato paste, 25
tomato sauce, 34–36
toppings: baked potatoes, 94–95; casseroles, 171, 177; popcorn, 90–91; soups, 34; yogurt, 84–85
tortillas, 65–67
tuna, 62–63

vegetables: casseroles, 169; fried rice, 163–66; frozen dumplings, 153–54; quesadillas, 66; ramen, 48; sandwiches, 63; sheet pan meals, 136–37; Sort-of Khao Soi, 161–63; stews, 30–31; stir-fry, 155–59

waffle cones, 178–79
wine, 38–39, 43

yogurt, 81–85

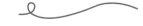

INDEX OF RECIPES

Acknowledgments

his book would simply not exist if it wasn't for Jess Zimmerman, a nimble editor and dear friend who punched up my jokes, tried out my weird ideas for bean salads, fielded after-hours text message meltdowns, and still had the capacity to come over and watch *Taskmaster* on my couch. Thank you, Jess, for convincing me to write this, and making sure I had fun doing it. Thank you to my excellent agent, Dana Murphy; I will play dice with you at an outdoor bar anytime. Big thanks to the entire team at Quirk Books.

I learned to order the thing that was most unusual to me on the menu from my dad, and that there is nothing wrong with putting a banana between two slices of bread and calling it a sandwich from my mom, both philosophies that fueled this book. Thank you, Mom and Dad. I love you, and please save me a slice of apple pie. Thanks to my wonderful brothers, Brendan and Conor, and my sisters-in-law, Susan and Lorianna, who have put up with so many of my culinary experiments, including, for Brendan, serving him a dandelion with sugar sprinkled on it in elementary school. (I'm sorry.) Thank you to the whole Brunner clan for their boundless love and enthusiasm, and to my terrific in-laws Helen, Don, Nina, and Chris.

So many of the ideas in this book came from bouncing around in the kitchen with my friends, dreaming up unhinged snack ideas. Thank you to my best friend of more than thirty-five years, Katie Porter, who suffered through a time of only eating salt-free Saltines. Thank you to fearless home cooking warriors Rachel Lowdermilk and Sam Roberts, who always bring joy and creativity into the kitchen. Thank you to the talented and kind Jett Allen for being an early reader, and a forever encourager. Thank you to my personal pastry scout and stylist-at-large Rachel Apatoff, a shiny gem of a human. Thank you to the many people who sent snacks and support throughout the process, particularly Jack Schmitz, Kelsey Youngman, Maia Murphy, Rachel Himmelfarb, Andrew Martin, Rupa Bhattacharya, Helena Fitzgerald, Emily Hughes, Helen Rosner, Kiki Aranita, Ari Miller, and Dayna Evans. Thank you to the brilliant writers, cooks, chefs, and recipe developers who inspired me and taught me how to feed myself when I didn't feel up to it. Thank you also to my therapist, and to the people who shore me up when I'm having a hard time with depression and anxiety.

Thank you most of all to my husband, Nick, for being my cheerleader, taster, proofreader, and partner in crime. I'll always save the last bit of blue cheese for you.

QUIRK BOOKS

David Borgenicht Chairman and Founder
Jhanteigh Kupihea President and Publisher
Nicole De Jackmo EVP, Deputy Publisher
Andie Reid Creative Director
Jane Morley Managing Editor
Mandy Sampson Production Director
Shaquona Crews Principal, Contracts and Rights
Katherine McGuire Assistant Director of Subsidiary Rights

CREATIVE

Alex Arnold Editorial Director, Children's
Jess Zimmerman Editor
Rebecca Gyllenhaal Associate Editor
Jessica Yang Assistant Editor

Elissa Flanigan Senior Designer
Paige Graff Junior Designer
Kassie Andreadis Managing Editorial Assistant

SALES, MARKETING, AND PUBLICITY

Kate Brown Senior Sales Manager
Christina Tatulli Digital Marketing Manager
Ivy Weir Senior Publicity and
Marketing Manager

Gaby Iori Publicist and Marketing Coordinator
Kim Ismael Digital Marketing Design Associate
Scott MacLean Publicity and
Marketing Assistant

OPERATIONS

Caprianna Anderson Business Associate
Robin Wright Production and Sales Assistant